Thrombosis and Inflammation in Acute Coronary Syndromes

Edited By

Ertugrul Ercan

Izmir University
Faculty of Medicine
Department of Cardiology Medicalpark Hospital
35000 Izmir-TURKEY

&

Gulfem Ece

Izmir University School of Medicine Medicalpark Hospital
Department of Medical Microbiology 35000 Izmir-TURKEY

General:

1. Any dispute or claim arising out of or in connection with this License Agreement or the Work (including non-contractual disputes or claims) will be governed by and construed in accordance with the laws of the U.A.E. as applied in the Emirate of Dubai. Each party agrees that the courts of the Emirate of Dubai shall have exclusive jurisdiction to settle any dispute or claim arising out of or in connection with this License Agreement or the Work (including non-contractual disputes or claims).

2. Your rights under this License Agreement will automatically terminate without notice and without the need for a court order if at any point you breach any terms of this License Agreement. In no event will any delay or failure by Bentham Science Publishers in enforcing your compliance with this License Agreement constitute a waiver of any of its rights.

3. You acknowledge that you have read this License Agreement, and agree to be bound by its terms and conditions. To the extent that any other terms and conditions presented on any website of Bentham Science Publishers conflict with, or are inconsistent with, the terms and conditions set out in this License Agreement, you acknowledge that the terms and conditions set out in this License Agreement shall prevail.

Bentham Science Publishers Ltd.
Executive Suite Y - 2
PO Box 7917, Saif Zone
Sharjah, U.A.E.
subscriptions@benthamscience.org

BENTHAM SCIENCE PUBLISHERS LTD.

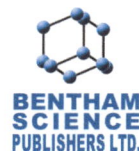

CONTENTS

Foreword   *i*

Preface   *iii*

List of Contributors   *vii*

CHAPTERS

1.	**Circulating Biomarkers of Vulnerable Atheromatous Plaques** *Xinkang Wang*	3
2.	**Tissue Factor Structure and Coagulation** *Jolanta Krudysz-Amblo, Kenneth G. Mann and Saulius Butenas*	23
3.	**Hemostasis: General Principles** *Melda Comert, Fahri Sahin and Guray Saydam*	59
4.	**Recurrent Thromboembolism** *Melda Comert, Guray Saydam and Fahri Sahin*	67
5.	**Antiplatelet Resistance** *Dilek Ural, İrem Yılmaz and Kurtuluş Karaüzüm*	79
6.	**Platelet Inhibitors for the Treatment of Acute Coronary Syndromes** *Hasan Gungor and Ceyhun Ceyhan*	105
7.	**Antiplatelet and Antithrombotic Therapy in Acute Coronary Syndrome in Patients with Chronic Kidney Disease** *Mahmut Altındal and Mustafa Arıcı*	121
8.	**Infectious Pathogens in Acute Atherosclerosis** *Gulfem Ece*	141
	Subject Index	153

FOREWORD

Atherosclerotic vascular disease is the leading cause of mortality in most parts of the world. Even with the most optimistic projections, it is expected to increase in the next decade. Although we have come a long way in preventing cardiovascular deaths, treating acute coronary syndromes and undertanding the biology of the disease, there is still much to learn. The accumulation of information in the field of thrombosis and atherosclerosis is immense. This book is a timely update on the new mechanisms and new approaches to treatment in the field. It is a useful resource to the clinician who wants to understand the mechanism and use the novel therapeutic approaches. An effort has been made to explain the basis of our therapeutic approaches. I hope this comprehensive book will be useful to the clinician.

Lale Tokgozoglu
Hacettepe University
Ankara
Turkey

PREFACE

This textbook covers many of the essential topics in the area of cardiovascular medicine. Pathophysiology of hemostasis and thrombosis are discussed extensively to make clear explanations for concepts behind thrombosis and heart disease. Mechanisms of thrombosis; the roles of cells, cytokines, and inflammation in the pathogenesis of cardiovascular diseases; and the evidence justifying current antithrombotic therapy are discussed under the light of latest multicenter, randomized clinical trials. Physiology, pathology and treatment of coronary artery thrombosis, the safety and efficacy of new heparins, direct thrombin inhibitors, glycoprotein IIb/IIIa inhibitors, new antiplatelet drugs, and new thrombolytic agents are mentioned. The coverage of trials focuses primarily on acute coronary syndromes. Coronary intervention (PCI) has become a well accepted therapy for stenotic coronary artery disease. Diagnostic and therapeutic interventions for coronary arterial disease are summarized with effective use of figures and tables. This book appeals to cardiologists, generalists, internists, family physicians, medical residents, and students. The emphasis are both practical and clinical. There are no heavy discussions of basic science or molecular mechanisms. Complex clinical trials are summarized but not dissected in detail.

Ertugrul Ercan
Izmir University
Faculty of Medicine
Department of Cardiology Medicalpark Hospital
35000 Izmir-Turkey

Gulfem Ece
Izmir University
School of Medicine
Medicalpark Hospital
Department of Medical Microbiology
35000 Izmir-Turkey

List of Contributors

Mahmut Altindal	Hacettepe University Faculty of Medicine, Department of Nephrology Ankara, Turkey
Jolanta Krudyszt Amblo	University of Vermont, Department of Biochemistry Burlington, Vermont, USA
Mustafa Arıcı	Hacettepe University Faculty of Medicine, Department of Nephrology Ankara, Turkey
Saulius Butenas	University of Vermont, Department of Biochemistry Burlington, Vermont, USA
Ceyhun Ceyhan	Adnan Menderes University School of Medicine Department of Cardiology, Aydin Turkey
Melda Comert	Ege University School of Medicine, Department of Hematology, Izmir, Turkey
Gulfem Ece	Izmir University School of Medicine, Medicalpark Hospital Department of Medical Microbiology, Izmir, Turkey
Ajda Gunes Ersoy	Ege University School of Medicine, Department of Hematology, Izmir, Turkey
Hasan Gungor	Adnan Menderes University School of Medicine, Department of Cardiology, Aydin, Turkey
Kurtulus Karauzum	Kocaeli University School of Medicine Department of Cardiology, Kocaeli, Turkey
Kenneth G. Mann	University of Vermont, Department of Biochemistry Burlington, Vermont, USA
Fahri Sahin	Ege University School of Medicine, Department of Hematology, Izmir, Turkey
Guray Saydam	Ege University School of Medicine, Department of Hematology, Izmir, Turkey
Dilek Ural	Kocaeli University School of Medicine Department of Cardiology, Kocaeli, Turkey
Xinkang Wang	Translational Science, Agennix Inc., Princeton,NJ 08540, USA
Irem Yilmaz	Kocaeli University School of Medicine Department of Cardiology, Kocaeli, Turkey

CHAPTER 1

Circulating Biomarkers of Vulnerable Atheromatous Plaques

Xinkang Wang[*]

Thrombosis Biology, Merck Research Laboratories, Kenilworth, NJ 07033, USA

Abstract: Rupture of atherosclerotic plaques is a major cause of cardiovascular events, including acute coronary syndromes, myocardial infarction and stroke. Identification of the vulnerable plaques is one of the most important steps leading to the treatment of patients with the disease. In spite of a considerable effort in identifying patients with vulnerable plaque, including the use of both circulatory and imaging biomarkers to delineate the molecular, cellular, and structural components and/or evolution of atherosclerosis and plaque vulnerability, it still lacks of such a specific biomarker for this disease. This review will focus on recent advances on discovery of circulating markers in atherosclerosis and hope that some of these markers might be of values to assess vulnerable atheromatous plaques. It is hoped that these biomarkers may be able to facilitate disease diagnosis and the development of new therapeutics to treat vulnerable plaque and its consequence of cardiovascular diseases.

Keywords: Atherosclerosis, atherosclerotic plaque, biomarker, cardiovascular disease, circulatory biomarker, inflammation, plaque rupture, translational medicine, vulnerable plaque.

INTRODUCTION: ATHEROSCLEROSIS AND VULNERABLE PLAQUE

Atherosclerosis is a major cause of cardiovascular disease, the top leading cause of morbidity and mortality in the United States [1] and the Western world. Atherosclerosis is the causative factor that leads to coronary artery disease (CAD, myocardial infarction and angina), peripheral vascular diseases (PAD, critical limb ischemia and intermittent claudication) and cerebral vascular disease (CVD, ischemic strokes). Atherosclerosis often occurs in medium and large arteries. It involves in a number of pathophysiological changes/features, including endothelial dysfunction, inflammation, and lipid deposits to form atherosclerotic "plaque" on the vessel wall [2, 3]. As the atheromatous plaque grows the vessel may undergo a remodeling to enlarge its dimension. Stenosis may occur when the

Corresponding author Xinkang Wang: Merck Research Laboratories, 2000 Galloping Hill Road, Kenilworth, NJ 07033, USA; Tel: 908-740-4879; E-mail: wangxk2000@yahoo.com

Ertugrul Ercan and Gulfem Ece (Eds.)

plaque makes up a significant portion of the intima and reduces the lumen, which restricts blood to flow through and reduces oxygen supply to the target organ. On the other hand, however, there is no direct correlation between stenosis and plaque vulnerability. For examples, approximately 30% patients with acute coronary syndrome (ACS) showed no significant stenotic plaques by angiography [4, 5]. Likewise, many patients with acute myocardial infarctions (AMI) triggered by occlusion of the coronary artery had no significant stenosis [6].

Atherosclerosis is a complex and progressive disease. The progression of the disease and composition of the plaque are influenced by inflammatory cells and the mediators they secrete. Atherosclerosis can also be affected by other risk factors such as hyperglycemia, elevated level of homocysteine, prothrombotic factors, as well as smoking. The interaction among inflammatory cells, vascular cells (such as endothelial cells and smooth muscle cells), various lipoproteins/particles, and many mediators lead to atherosclerotic plaque development.

Atherosclerosis process is thought to be initiated with the infiltration of inflammatory cells through the compromised endothelium to become subendothelial macrophages, which accumulate cholesterol to form foam cells and then form fatty streak [2, 3]. The atherosclerotic lesion develops (becomes an intermediate lesion) over time when smooth muscle cells migrate into the subendothelium, proliferate, and lay down extracellular matrix to form the fibrous cap. The atherosclerotic lesion further grows and evolves with the participation of various risk factors (such as high levels of LDL, inflammation, shear and oxidative stresses) and various cell components (such as macrophages, T cells and smooth muscle cells) [2, 3]. The stability of atheroma is known to be associated with the thickness of the fibrous cap, which can be modified by matrix metalloproteinase (MMP) activities, and may ultimately lead to plaque erosion, rupture, and thrombosis for vascular occlusion [7, 8]. The rate of atherosclerosis progression leading to plaque rupture/erosion and vessel occlusion in patients is still unknown.

Most of our current knowledge regarding vulnerable atheromatous plaque is based on retrospective histopathological studies of postmortem specimens, of which distinct composition and characteristics for high-risk/vulnerable plaques are suggested, including a thin fibrous cap, a large lipid-rich core and increased macrophage activity [2-5, 7, 8]. Recent advances in molecular and structural imaging and circulatory risk factors have provided a better understanding of the mechanisms of atherosclerosis development and insights on plaques prone to rupture and/or erosion [9, 10].

BIOMARKERS IN ATHEROSCLEROSIS

Biomarkers are defined by the NIH working group as "a characteristic that is objectively measured and evaluated as an indicator of normal biological processes, pathogenic processes or pharmacological responses to a therapeutic intervention" [11]. A biomarker may be measured in blood, urine or a tissue, or may be a recording of a process. It is critical that the biological variables are measured quantitatively and with acceptable reproducibility, sensitivity and specificity. A biomarker can be used to monitor disease progression, target engagement, pharmacokinetics and pharmacodynamics (both efficacy and safety) correlation, as well as patient selection and stratification [12].

Two major biomarker strategies that have been extensively used in atherosclerosis research, including (1) imaging biomarker strategies for the structural and molecular components of plaque, such as magnetic resonance imaging, computed tomography, positron emission tomography, ultrasound, and optical imaging to study the thin fibrous cap, necrotic core, plaque inflammation, neovascularization, intra-plaque hemorrhage and calcification, and (2) circulatory biomarker strategy for various risk factors in blood samples. Since the primary focus of this chapter is on those of circulating biomarkers, imaging biomarkers for the assessment of vulnerable atherosclerotic plaques have only been briefly summarized in the last section.

CIRCULATING BIOMARKERS FOR VULNERABLE ATHEROMATOUS PLAQUES

Atherosclerotic plaque contains a large number of inflammatory cells and dysfunctional vascular cells (such as smooth muscle cells and endothelial cells), as well as mediators that they secrete or microparticles that they derive. These mediators and microparticles released into circulation may reflect the pathology of the atheromatous plaque (such as inflammation, endothelial damage), or change of hemostasis for cardiovascular risk and plaque vulnerability. While many remain be validated, these circulatory biomarkers may be of value to correlate with plaque vulnerability. Representatives of promising circulatory biomarkers for vulnerable atheromatous plaque are summarized in Table **1** [13-56], including non-specific inflammatory biomarkers, inflammatory cytokines and mediators, extracellular mediators, atherosclerosis-related and atherothrombosis-related biomarkers, and other circulatory biomarkers.

Table 1: Representative Circulating Biomarkers for Vulnerable Atheromatous Plaque

Marker	Function	Clinical impotance	References
Non-Specific Inflammatory Biomarkers			
CRP	A circulatory protein that binds to phosphocholine on the surface of dead/dying cells and to activate the complement system	CRP is one of the best characterized inflammatory markers, and has been shown its value as a CHD biomarker.	[13, 14]
MPO	A peroxidase enzyme most abundantly expressed in neutrophil granulocytes	MPO possesses potent proinflammatory properties ad may directly contribute to tissue injury. Serum MPO was shown to predict risk in patients with ACS and chest pain.	[15, 16]
Inflammatory Cytokines, Chemokines, and Adhesion Molecules			
IL-6	A pleiotropic cytokine plays an important role in immune and inflammatory responses	IL-6 is associated with the development of atherosclerosis. Elevated levels of serum IL-6 were associated with plaque stability in carotid disease and CHD patients.	[17, 18]
IL-18	A cytokine plays an important role in cell-mediated immune responses	Elevated serum levels of IL-18 were considered as a strong independent predictor of cardiovascular death in patients with CAD.	[19, 20]
TNFa	A cytokine involved in systemic inflammation	TNFa is involved in atherosclerotic progression. Plasma levels of TNFa were significantly increased in patients with unstable plaques.	[21]
CXCR1/CXCR2	Closely related receptors for IL-8	CXCR1 and CXCR2 are activated by IL-8 to induce leukocyte recruitment and activation at sites of inflammation. Elevated levels of CXCR1 and CXCR2 were observed in peripheral blood cells in patients with obstructive CAD.	[22]
sVCAM-1	A soluable form of VCAM-1 protein that mediates the adhesion of leukocytes to vascular endothelium	VCAM-1 mediates the adhesion of leukocytes to vascular endothelium. It may play a role in the development of atherosclerosis. Evaluated levels of sVCAM-1 were observed in CAD patients.	[23, 24]
sICAM-1	A soluable form of ICAM-1 protein that mediates keukocyte-endothelial cell-cell interactions and leukocyte transmigration	ICAM-1 mediates the adhesion of leukocytes to vascular endothelium. It may play a role in the development of atherosclerosis. Evaluated levels of sICAM-1 were observed in CAD patients.	[23, 24]
sE-selectin	A soluable form of a cell adhesion molecule expressed only on endothelial cells for leukocytes	E-selectin mediates the adhesion of leukocytes to vascular endothelium. It may play a role in the development of atherosclerosis. Evaluated levels of sE-selectin were observed in CAD patients.	[23, 24]
sP-selectin	A soluable form of a cell adhesion molecule plays a role in the initial recruitment of leukocytes to the site of injury during inflammation	P-selectin expressed on activated endothelial cells and is involved in the initial recruitment of leukocytes to the injury during inflammation. Evaluated levels of sP-selectin were observed in CAD patients.	[23, 24]
sCD40L	A pleiotropic immunomodulator	CD40L is primarily expressed on activateds T-cells and platelets. It binds to CD40. sCD40L is a marker of platelet activation and an independent predictor of outcome in ACS.	[25, 26]
Extracellular Mediators			
MMP9	A protease of the MMP family involved in the breakdown of extracellular matrix	MMP-9 is involved in atherosclerotic plaque development. Higher levels of MMP-9 were shown to be associated with destabilization of the plaque in CAD patients.	[27-30]
Osteopontin	An extracellular protein with multifunctions, including inhibits vascular calcification	Elevated serum levels of OPN are associated with carotid plaque stability in patients and in response to statin treatment.	[31, 32]

Table 1: contd….

Osteoprotegerin	A decoy receptor for the receptor activator of nuclear factor kappa B ligand (RANKL) and to inhibit nuclear kappa B (NF-κB) activities	Elevated serum levels of OPN are associated with carotid plaque stability in patients and in response to statin treatment.	[31, 32]
Atherosclerosis-Related Biomarkers			
Lp-PLA2	A secreted enzyme that catalyzes the degradation of platelet-activating factor	Lp-PLA2 is involved in the development of atherosclerosis. Significantly elevated plasma levels and activity of Lp-PLA2 were observed in patients with CAD and ischemic stroke risk.	[33-35]
Oxidized LDL	An oxidized form of LDL particles that transport fat molecules and cholesterol into the vessel wall	Oxidized LDL plays a central role in initiation and progression of atherosclerosis. Elevated levels of oxidized LDL showed strong corelation with CHD events.	[36-38]
sCD36	A soluble form of the transmembrane glycoprotein expressed in a variety of tissues and cells	CD36 is involved in inflammation and the development of atherosclerosis. Plasma levels of sCD36 were elevated in CAD patients.	[39]
Atherothrombosis-Related Biomarkers			
VWF	A blood glycoprotein produced by endothelial cells and involved in hemostasis	VWF is a well-established marker of endothelial damage and dysfunction and contributes to platelet adhesion. Elevated levels of plasma VWF were observed in CAD patients.	[40-42]
Tissue Factor	A protein present in subendothelial tissue and leukocytes necessary for the initiation of thrombin formation	TF plays a key role in activation of the extrinsic coagulation pathway to tiger thrombus formation. High circulating levels of TF were associated with ACS in patients.	[43, 44]
Microparticles	Fragments derived from stimulated or apoptotic cells by plasma membrane remodeling	High levels of microparticles are found in both atherosclerotic plaques and in circulation. Circulating microparticles may be associated with thrombus formation during plaque rupture.	[45-47]
Other Biomarkers			
Adiponectin	An insulin-sensitizing plasma protein expressed in adipose tissue	Adiponectin is known to have a protective role against atherogenesis. Reduced plasma levels of adiponectin wwere found in patients with CAD risk.	[48-53]
HSP-27	A shaperone molecule	Hsp27 provides thermotolerance in vivo, cytoprotection, and support of cell survival under stress conditions. Plasma levels of HSP-27 were significantly decreased in CAD patients.	[54]
Troponin	A protein complex contributed to skeletal and cardiac muscle contraction	Cardiac troponins (cTn) are released into the circulation during cardiomyocyte injury, thus the serum levels of cTn might be a diagnostic marker for atherosclerotic burden in ACS patients.	[55, 56]

Non-Specific Inflammatory Biomarkers

Complement Reactive Protein

Complement reactive protein (CRP), a member of the pentraxin family, is the most extensively studied inflammatory and coronary heart disease (CHD) biomarker [57]. An increase in CRP levels is common in both infectious and non-infectious disorders. Large clinical studies provided positive associations between the carotid intima-media thickness (CIMT, an imaging biomarker that has been extensively used to measure atherosclerotic plaque) and plasma levels of CRP [58], suggesting a potential utility of CRP in identifying patients at high risk of atherosclerotic complications [13]. Further studies after statin therapy suggest that CRP may serve as a CAD risk marker and therapeutic intervention [14], showing potential correlation with LDL [59, 60]. Other studies, however, were inconclusive regarding a causal role of CRP in CHD [61], which is also supported by a genome-wide association study on CRP gene with CHD [62]. In addition, CRP is considered more as a general inflammatory marker than a specific one in atherosclerosis because it can be derived from multiple sources throughout the body and elevated in many disease states. Overall, the role of CRP as a specific predictor of CAD remains to be validated [57, 63-65].

Myeloperoxidase

Myeloperoxidase (MPO) is a hemoprotein produced by polymorphonuclear neutrophils and macrophages and secreted during activation. MPO possesses potent proinflammatory properties and may directly contribute to tissue injury. MPO also has been linked to the development of lipid-laden soft plaque, the activation of protease cascades affecting the stability of plaque, the production of cytotoxic and prothrombogenic oxidized lipids, and the consumption of nitric oxide leading to vasoconstriction [66, 67]. Serum MPO concentration was shown to predict risk in patients with ACS and chest pain [15, 16]. Similarly, high levels of serum MPO were significantly elevated in patients with ACS presenting with eroded culprit plaque compared with patients presenting with ruptured culprit plaque [68]. Thus, MPO has been proposed as a marker of plaque instability even if it is not specific to cardiac diseases. Another report however argued that the serum MPO level might be independent of the commonly measured risk factors of atherosclerosis [69].

Inflammatory Cytokines, Chemokines, and Adhesion Molecules

Cytokines, chemokines, and adhesion molecules play a critical role in vascular inflammation, atheroma formation and complication. Several of these inflammatory cytokines, such as interleukin (IL)-6, IL-18, tumor necrosis factor-α (TNF-α), chemokines and chemokine receptors, and adhesion molecules present in both atherosclerotic plaques and the systemic circulation, and are associated with the progression and stability of atherosclerotic plaques.

Interleukin-6

IL-6 is a pleiotropic cytokine in immune and inflammatory responses. IL-6 is associated with the development of atherosclerosis. The level of IL- 6 expression was elevated on the site of coronary plaque rupture [70] and in cardiovascular events [71]. The levels of IL-6 were markedly increased at the plaque site and the high levels of local release were associated with lower plaque echogenicity in patients subjected to carotid artery stenting [17], suggesting a possible correlation between inflammation and plaque stability. Likewise, the MONIC/KORA study showed elevated levels of both CRP and IL-6 in CHD patients [18]. Like CRP, the reality of IL-6 as a specific biomarker of vulnerable plaques remains to be vigorously validated.

Interleukin-18

IL-18 is a pleiotropic proinflammatory cytokine produced by monocytes and macrophages, and plays an important role in cell-mediated immune responses. Increased expression of IL-18 was observed in atherosclerotic plaques, especially in those prone to rupture based on assessment of endarterectomy specimens [72]. However, Abe *et al.*, [17] showed that the local levels of IL-18 at the plaque site only slightly increased in patients subjected to carotid artery stenting. Elevated serum levels of IL-18 were considered as a strong independent predictor of cardiovascular death in patients with CAD [19], and might be associated with accelerated vulnerability of atherosclerotic plaques. Since conflict outcomes are noted for the significance of the association of elevated levels of IL-18 with CHD risk [19, 20], the prognostic value of plasma IL-18 for atherothrombotic events remains to be further evaluated.

Tumor Necrosis Factor-α

TNFα is a pleiotropic pro-inflammatory cytokine secreted by various cells including activated monocytes, macrophages, lymphocytes, adipocytes, and various vascular cells. TNFα is involved in atherosclerotic progression from the initial stage of plaque formation, to plaque progression,and ultimately to plaque erosion/rupture and vessel occlusion. Circulating levels of TNFα, along with MMPs and IL-8 were significantly increased in patients with unstable plaques than those of stable lesions [21], suggesting that circulating TNFα might be a biomarker of vulnerable plaques. Similar to IL-6 and IL-18, the use of TNFα as a specific biomarker of vulnerable plaque remains to be validated.

Chemokines and Chemokine Receptors

Chemokines are inflammatory cytokines characterized by their ability to cause directed migration of leukocytes into atherosclerotic plaques. Elevated expression of chemokines, IL-8, neutrophil-activating peptide-2, interferon-γ-inducible protein 10, monocyte chemoattractant protein-1, and leukotactin-1 in atherosclerotic lesions has been demonstrated [73]. Combined measurements of multiple chemokines might be of more value as a "signature of disease" to serve as an accurate method to assess for the presence of atherosclerotic disease [73]. Similarly, mRNA expression array to identify significant increases in IL-8 and its receptors such as CXCR1 and CXCR2 in peripheral blood cells in patients with obstructive CAD [22] could be of biomarker value for vulnerable plaques.

Soluble Adhesion Molecules

Adhesion Molecules Adhesion molecules play an important role in the development of atherosclerosis. Levels of soluble adhesion molecules, including soluble vascular cellular adhesion molecule-1 (sVCAM-1), soluble intercellular adhesion molecule-1 (sICAM-1) and soluble E-selectin (sE-selectin), were associated with increased risk of cardiovascular death in CAD patients [23]. Evaluated levels of soluble adhesion molecules (such as sVCAM-1, sE-selectin and sP-selectin) were observed in patients with various clinical presentations of coronary atherosclerosis, suggesting potential association of soluble adhesion molecules and inflammation with coronary plaque destabilization [24]. In addition, membrane-shed microparticles isolated from human atherosclerotic plaques were found to be able to transfer ICAM-1 to endothelial cells to recruit inflammatory cells and thus the possibly to promote plaque progression [74]. Furthermore, while the value of soluble adhesion molecules as a biomarker for vulnerable plaque remains to be validated, molecular imaging targeting specific endothelial adhesion molecules may provide insights into atherosclerosis development.

Circulating Soluble CD40 Ligand

Circulating soluble CD40 ligand (sCD40L) is a pleiotropic immunomodulator. sCD40L and its receptor (CD40) are expressed by endothelial cells, smooth muscle cells, monocytes/macrophages, T-cells and platelets. Both CD40 and CD40L are present in human atherosclerotic lesions [75]. CD40-CD40L interactions mediate several of the processes that set the stage for plaque rupture, like degradation of the extracellular matrix and formation of the necrotic core, and trigger the expression of other inflammatory and proatherogenic mediators [76]. Mice deficient in CD40L had less atherosclerosis and stabilized the atherosclerotic plaques, with features of low in inflammation and high in fibrosis [77-80]. Elevated plasma levels of sCD40L have been observed in patients with ACS in the CAPTURE study [25] and FRISC study [26]. Also, a single nucleotide polymorphism was been demonstrated the benefit in the CD40L gene from the FRISC study and revealed a correlation between elevated sCD40L levels and a prothrombotic state [26]. In contrast, the Dallas Heart

Study showed no association of sCD40L with most atherosclerosis risk factors or with subclinical atherosclerosis [81], raising a question about the utility of sCD40L in screening for high risk patients.

Extracellular Mediators and Biomarkers

Matrix Metalloproteinases

MMPs are a family of zinc- and calcium-dependent endopeptidases that play a key role in the regulation of extracellular matrix formation and stability with a strong influence on arterial wall remodeling. For example, MMP-9 was found to be involved in degradation of the matrix surrounding smooth muscle cells and facilitating smooth muscle cell migration [82]. Growing evidence suggests a strong relationship between MMPs and atherosclerotic plaque instability and consequent cardiovascular events [8]. Elevated levels of MMPs were shown in both atherosclerotic plaques and circulation. Plasma MMP-8 levels were significantly elevated in patients with unstable angina [83] and with carotid atherosclerosis [84]. Similarly, both plasma active MMP-3 and active MMP-9 were independently associated with history of in-stent restenosis [85]. Furthermore, higher levels of MMP-9 were shown to be associated with destabilization of the plaque [27], and MMP-9 serum concentrations were associated with CAD [28, 29] and with unstable carotid plaques [23]. Plasma MMP-9, along with multiple plasma biomarkers, was significantly higher in patients with ruptured plaques, but the measurement of these biomarkers was incapable of predicting the presence of vulnerable plaque determined by virtual histology intravascular ultrasound [30]. While it remains to be further validated, these evidences support for an important role of multiple MMPs and possibly tissue inhibitor of metalloproteinases (TIMPs) in plaque destabilization and rupture. In addition to the direct measurement of circulating MMPs, the MMP activity in the atherosclerotic plaque could also be monitored by molecular imaging *in vivo* [86].

Osteopontin and Osteoprotegerin

Osteopontin (OPN) is a multifunctional protein, highly expressed in bone and also expressed by various cell types including macrophages, endothelial cells, smooth muscle cells in the vessel wall. Osteoprotegerin (OPG) is a secretory glycoprotein that belongs to the tumor necrosis factor receptor family. OPG is produced by a variety of tissues, including bones and the cardiovascular system (heart, arteries and veins). OPN and OPG are known vascular calcification inhibitors, which were demonstrated to be correlated with inflammation and cardiovascular events. Both OPG and OPN are upregulated in symptomatic human carotid atherosclerosis with possible implications for plaque stability [87]. The elevated serum OPN and OPG levels in patients with carotid stenosis had independent association between these biochemical markers, the gray-scale median (GSM; a tool in selecting patients for carotid artery stenting) score and carotid-induced symptomatology. Therefore, these bone-matrix proteins combined with GSM could be potential markers for vulnerable carotid plaques [31]. Furthermore, serum OPN and OPG are sensitive markers for statin-treatment response in carotid plaque stabilization [32].

Atherosclerosis-Related Biomarkers

Lipoprotein-Associated Phospholipase A$_2$

Lipoprotein-associated phospholipase A2 (Lp-PLA2) is a 50-kDa calcium-insensitive lipase produced predominantly by macrophages and lymphocytes. This enzyme resides mainly in LDL particles in plasma. Significantly elevated plasma levels and activity of Lp-PLA2 were observed in patients with CAD and ischemic stroke risk [33-35]. The activity of Lp-PLA2 is also associated with the progress of atherosclerosis and plaque rupture [88]. While both pro- and anti-inflammatory activities have been demonstrated for Lp-PLA2, its primary role in atherosclerosis appears to be pro-atherogenic, in part due to its role in hydrolyzing oxidized phospholipids, generating proinflammatory moieties lysophosphatidylcholine and oxidized fatty acids [35, 86]. Evidence supporting the importance of Lp-PLA$_2$ in atherosclerosis includes its localization in the atherosclerotic lesions, in particular within the necrotic core and in macrophages, notably apoptotic macrophages, surrounding vulnerable and ruptured plaques in patients who suffered from sudden coronary death [89]. Since Lp-PLA$_2$ is an independent predictor of risk, it may be superior to inflammatory biomarkers for atherosclerosis. Inhibition of Lp-PLA$_2$ was demonstrated to reduce complex coronary atherosclerotic plaque development in swine and in patients [90, 91]. It is still not clear, however, if Lp-PLA$_2$ acts as a true biological effector of cardiovascular diseases or as useful biomarker of the disease severity such as plaque rupture [35].

Oxidized Low-Density Lipoprotein

Oxidized low-density lipoprotein (LDL) plays a central role in initiation and progression of atherosclerosis. Oxidized LDL is associated with a number of pathophysiological events in atherosclerosis development, including endothelial cell dysfunction, leukocyte recruitment, foam cell formation, and plaque transition from stable to unstable/vulnerable conditions. It was postulated that oxidized LDL may also promote the progress of atherosclerosis by acting through its toxic effects on stem cells that participate in vascular damage repairing including inflammatory injury of atherosclerosis [92]. Elevated plasma levels of oxidized

LDL were observed in patients with ACS [36, 93] and shown to be the strongest predictor of CHD events compared with a conventional lipoprotein profile and other traditional risk factors for CHD [37]. Interestingly, among several oxidative stress markers investigated in human carotid plaques, only oxidized LDL was significantly increased and associated with clinical symptoms [94]. In spite of strong evidence that circulating oxidized LDL levels correlate independently with various forms of coronary and peripheral arterial disease [38], it remains to be validated if oxidized LDL is a useful biomarker to differentiate various stages of atherosclerosis including plaque instability.

Soluble CD36

CD36 is a transmembrane glycoprotein expressed in a variety of tissues and has been shown to be involved in atherosclerosis, angiogenesis, inflammation, lipid metabolism and platelet activation. CD36 was localized to macrophage-rich area of intima within the atherosclerotic lesion [95]. Membrane CD36 in monocytes and macrophages is upregulated by oxidized LDL and involved in the differentiation of macrophages into foam cells [96]. Plasma levels of soluble CD36 (sCD36) were increased in patients with symptomatic atherosclerotic carotid plaques and is related to plaque stability, suggesting that sCD36 could be a marker of plaque instability [39]. A recent report showed that sCD36 was significantly associated with indices of insulin resistance, carotid atherosclerosis and fatty liver in a nondiabetic healthy population [95].

Atherothrombosis-Related Biomarkers

von Willebrand Factor

von Willebrand factor (VWF) plays a pivotal role in platelet adhesion and aggregation at sites of high shear. VWF is a well-established marker for endothelial damage and dysfunction. VWF is prominently present at the site of platelet accumulation in coronary thrombi, suggesting that it is not only a marker but also a mediator of cardiovascular disease events [40]. VWR plasma levels were associated with CIMT and a marker of vascular damage, urinary microalbumin excretion [41]. VWF is a significantly increased in patients with ACS [40]. A later study showed, however, that Japanese as compared to white Americans had similar levels of D-dimer and higher levels of VWF although Japanese had a significantly lower prevalence of coronary artery calcification (CAC, a risk factor of atherosclerosis and plaque vulnerability) and CIMT [42], suggesting that VWF as a biomarker of vulnerable plaque remains to be validated.

Tissue Factor

Tissue factor (TF) plays a key role in activation of the extrinsic coagulation pathway to tiger thrombus formation. TF is one of the main proteins that may link proinflammatory and prothrombotic processes for atherosclerotic development and plaque rupture [97]. Three distinct pools of circulating TF have been identified, including TF-bearing microparticles, cell-associated TF, and soluble alternative splicing TF (asTF) [43, 44, 98]. TF-bearing microparticles are derived from apoptotic cells such as macrophages, smooth muscle cells and endothelium. Cell-associated TF is located on cell surface of leukocytes and platelets. Soluble asTF is generated by alternative splicing of its full-length mRNA [43, 44, 98]. All three forms of TF might be associated with thrombus growth. High levels of circulating TF are associated with the formation of a larger or more stable thrombus, and more severe ACS, suggesting that circulating TF may represent a useful biomarker for patients with a high-risk profile of developing major cardiovascular events [43, 44]. While circulating TF may contribute to the hypercoagulable state of the blood, its value as a biomarker of plaque rupture and atherothrombosis remains to be validated.

Microparticles

Microparticles are fragments released from stimulated or apoptotic cells by plasma membrane remodeling. High levels of microparticles are found in both atherosclerotic plaques and in circulation [45]. Microparticles can be derived from monocytes, lymphocytes, smooth muscle cells and endothelial cells, as well as platelets, and retained considerable levels of TF activity [45, 46]. Plaque microparticles favor local inflammation by augmenting adhesion molecule expression at the surface of endothelial cell and facilitating monocyte recruitment. Plaque microparticles also stimulate intraplaque angiogenesis and promote local cell apoptosis [45], and contribute to plaque progression and rupture. Circulating microparticles impair the atheroprotective function of the vascular endothelium and promote thrombus formation in the event of plaque rupture. Circulating microparticles are elevated in patients with atherothrombotic diseases [45, 47] and may serve as a useful biomarker of vascular injury and a potential predictor of CAD.

Other Biomarkers

Adiponectin

Adiponectin is an insulin-sensitizing plasma protein expressed in adipose tissue and has also been suggested to play a role in atherosclerosis and cardiovascular disease [48]. The protective role of adiponectin against atherogenesis might be mediated through acting on the endothelium and smooth muscle cells, raising NO secretion and inhibiting production of adhesion factors [49]. Adiponectin inhibits monocyte adhesion and phagocytic activity, and further suppresses the accumulation of modified lipoproteins of form cells in the vascular wall [50]. Adiponectin is reduced in obesity and type 2 diabetes, and hypoadiponectinemia has been associated with increased risk of CAD and ACS in several but not all clinical studies [51]. For examples, low plasma adiponection levels were found to be associated with presence of thin-cap fibroatheroma in men with stable CAD [52] and correlated with increased CIMT in a multiethnic cohort [53], supporting a protective role for adiponectin in atherosclerosis. Further studies are needed, however, to clarify the relevance of adiponectin as a specific biomarker of vulnerable plaque and in response to treatment.

Serum Heat-Shock Protein 27

Serum Heat-Shock Protein 27 (HSP27) is a molecular chaperone involved in different processes, including stress response, apoptosis, cell differentiation, and modulation of the actin cytoskeleton. Decreased levels of HSP27 were observed in patients with cardiovascular diseases, and serum concentration of HSP27 was significantly inversely correlated to CIMT [54], suggesting that it might be a useful circulatory biomarker for cardiovascular events. While it remains to be further validated, HSP27 could not be a specific marker for plaque vulnerability due to its broad spectrum of biological activities.

Troponins (Tn)

Troponin is a complex of three regulatory proteins (troponin C, troponin I and troponin T) that contribute to the contraction of skeletal and cardiac muscle. Cardiac troponins (cTn) are released into the circulation during cardiomyocyte injury and might be used as a diagnostic marker for various heart disorders such as myocardial infarction and ACS [55, 56]. Recent introduction of high sensitive cardiac troponin T (hs-cTnT) assays may provide diagnostic values for quantitative assessment of coronary atherosclerotic plaque burden and ACS [55, 56].

IMAGING BIOMARKERS FOR VULNERABLE ATHEROMATOUS PLAQUES

In addition to the circulatory biomarkers, various imaging biomarkers, both invasive and noninvasive imaging modalities, have been demonstrated a considerable value for the diagnosis of atherosclerosis disease progression and/or in response to treatments. Applications of these imaging biomarkers in atherosclerosis have been extensively reviewed [99-106]. Invasive imaging, such as intravascular ultrasound (IVUS), intravascular optical coherence tomography (OCT) and intravascular MRI, provides advantages for its close assessment of atherosclerotic lesion due to probe miniaturization and very close to the plaque. A recent PROSPECT (Providing Regional Observations to Study Predictors of Events in the Coronary Tree) study provided an excellent example for the use of IVUS in high-risk atherosclerotic plaque patients and its great correlation with the possibility to cause cardiac events [107]. In contrast, noninvasive imaging provides considerable flexibility and advantages to assess not only the plaque morphology but also the molecular/cellar events upon application of specific contrast agents targeting molecules of interest in the plaque. For example, MRI is useful to assess plaque burden, remodeling and lipid-rich core; MRI with dynamic contrast-enhanced gadolinium (DCE-Gd) may allow to study the plaque inflammation and neovascularization [103, 105]. Other noninvasive imaging modalities such as PET imaging using [18F] fluorodeoxyglucose (FDG) may provide assessment of inflammatory activity in the plaque [104, 108]. In particular, many radiolabelled probes have been developed for detecting atherosclerotic unstable plaques by means of nuclear imaging techniques like PET and SPECT [104]. Overall, with recent advances in both imaging technologies and the development of imaging contrast agents, imaging biomarkers have provided great promise to facilitate the assessment of vulnerable plaques.

CONCLUSION

While a number of circulating biomarkers showed some promise of their value to assess high risk plaques, none is qualified as a surrogate biomarker to date. Since atherosclerosis is a complex disease and many factors contribute to the disease progression and plaque rupture, multi-biomarkers represent the cardiovascular risks may be considered to predict vulnerable atheromatous plaques, including those existed *in situ* for plaque instability, such as cytokines, MMPs and plaque microparticles and their activities, and those elevated/altered in the circulation. Likewise, a combination of multiple circulatory biomarkers with various mechanisms as described in this chapter might be used as a signature of the disease and plaque vulnerability. In addition, the combination of circulatory biomarkers with imaging biomarkers, in particular with molecular imaging, which not only allow to monitor the structure but also the molecular and cellular components of the plaque development [99-106], may provide a greater hope to predict plaque rupture and/or to investigate responses to therapeutic intervention of CAD.

ACKNOWLEDGEMENTS

Declared none.

CONFLICT OF INTEREST

The authors confirm that this chapter contents have no conflict of interest.

REFERENCES

[1]   American Heart Association. Statistics. http://www.americanheart.org/ (Accessed April 2012).
[2]   Ross R. Atherosclerosis--an inflammatory disease. N Engl J Med 1999; 340: 115-26.
[3]   Libby P. Vascular biology of atherosclerosis: overview and state of the art. Am J Cardiol 2003; 91: 3A-6A.
[4]   Kullo IJ, Edwards WD, Schwartz RS. Vulnerable plaque: pathobiology and clinical implications. Ann Intern Med 1998; 129: 1050-60.
[5]   Kolodgie FD, Burke AP, Farb A, *et al*. The thin-cap fibroatheroma: a type of vulnerable plaque: the major precursor lesion to acute coronary syndromes. Curr Opin Cardiol 2001; 16: 285-92.
[6]   Ambrose JA, Fuster V. The risk of coronary occlusion is not proportional to the prior severity of coronary stenoses. Heart 1998; 79: 3-4.
[7]   Naghavi M, Libby P, Falk E, *et al*. From vulnerable plaque to vulnerable patient: a call for new definitions and risk assessment strategies: Part I. Circulation 2003; 108: 1664-72.
[8]   Toutouzas K, Synetos A, Nikolaou C, Tsiamis E, Tousoulis D, Stefanadis C. Matrix metalloproteinases and vulnerable atheromatous plaque. Curr Top Med Chem 2012.
[9]   Schaar JA, Muller JE, Falk E, *et al*. Terminology for high-risk and vulnerable coronary artery plaques. Report of a meeting on the vulnerable plaque, June 17 and 18, 2003, Santorini, Greece. Eur Heart J 2004; 25: 1077-82.
[10]   Virmani R, Kolodgie FD, Burke AP, Farb A, Schwartz SM. Lessons from sudden coronary death: a comprehensive morphological classification scheme for atherosclerotic lesions. Arterioscler Thromb Vasc Biol 2000; 20: 1262-75.
[11]   Biomarkers Definitions Working Group. Biomarkers and surrogate endpoints: preferred definitions and conceptual framework. Clin Pharmacol Ther 2001; 69: 89-95.
[12]   Feuerstein GZ, Dormer C, Ruffolo RR Jr., Stiles G, Walsh FL, Rutkowski LJ, Translational medicine perspectives of biomarkers in drug discovery and development: Part I Target selection and validation. Am Drug Discovery, 2007; 5: 36-43.
[13]   Ridker PM, Brown NJ, Vaughan DE, Harrison DG, Mehta JL. Established and emerging plasma biomarkers in the prediction of first atherothrombotic events. Circulation 2004; 109: IV6-19.
[14]   Ridker PM, Cannon CP, Morrow D, *et al*. C-reactive protein levels and outcomes after statin therapy. N Engl J Med 2005; 352: 20-8.
[15]   Baldus S, Heeschen C, Meinertz T, *et al*. Myeloperoxidase serum levels predict risk in patients with acute coronary syndromes. Circulation 2003; 108: 1440-5.
[16]   Brennan ML, Penn MS, Van Lente F, *et al*. Prognostic value of myeloperoxidase in patients with chest pain. N Engl J Med 2003; 349: 1595-604.
[17]   Abe Y, Sakaguchi M, Furukado S, *et al*. Associations of local release of inflammatory biomarkers during carotid artery stenting with plaque echogenicity and calcification. Cerebrovasc Dis 2010; 30: 402-9.
[18]   Koenig W, Khuseyinova N, Baumert J, *et al*. Increased concentrations of C-reactive protein and IL-6 but not IL-18 are independently associated with incident coronary events in middle-aged men and women: results from the MONICA/KORA Augsburg case-cohort study, 1984-2002. Arterioscler Thromb Vasc Biol 2006; 26: 2745-51.
[19]   Blankenberg S, Tiret L, Bickel C, *et al*. Interleukin-18 is a strong predictor of cardiovascular death in stable and unstable angina. Circulation 2002; 106: 24-30.

[20]   Blankenberg S, Luc G, Ducimetière P, *et al.* Interleukin-18 and the risk of coronary heart disease in European men: the Prospective Epidemiological Study of Myocardial Infarction (PRIME). Circulation 2003; 108: 2453-9.

[21]   Pelisek J, Rudelius M, Zepper P, *et al.* Multiple biological predictors for vulnerable carotid lesions. Cerebrovasc Dis 2009; 28: 601-10.

[22]   Leonard DA, Merhige ME, Williams BA, Greene RS. Elevated expression of the interleukin-8 receptors CXCR1 and CXCR2 in peripheral blood cells in obstructive coronary artery disease. Coron Artery Dis 2011; 22: 491-6.

[23]   Blankenberg S, Rupprecht HJ, Bickel C, *et al.* Circulating cell adhesion molecules and death in patients with coronary artery disease. Circulation 2001; 104: 1336-42.

[24]   Guray U, Erbay AR, Guray Y, *et al.* Levels of soluble adhesion molecules in various clinical presentations of coronary atherosclerosis. Int J Cardiol 2004; 96: 235-40.

[25]   Heeschen C, Dimmeler S, Hamm CW, *et al.* Soluble CD40 ligand in acute coronary syndromes. N Engl J Med 2003; 348: 1104-11.

[26]   Malarstig A, Lindahl B, Wallentin L, Siegbahn A. Soluble CD40L levels are regulated by the -3459 A>G polymorphism and predict myocardial infarction and the efficacy of antithrombotic treatment in non-ST elevation acute coronary syndrome. Arterioscler Thromb Vasc Biol 2006; 26: 1667-73.

[27]   Morishige K, Shimokawa H, Matsumoto Y, *et al.* Overexpression of matrix metalloproteinase-9 promotes intravascular thrombus formation in porcine coronary arteries in vivo. Cardiovasc Res 2003; 57: 572-85.

[28]   Noji Y, Kajinami K, Kawashiri MA, *et al.* Circulating matrix metalloproteinases and their inhibitors in premature coronary atherosclerosis. Clin Chem Lab Med 2001; 39: 380-4.

[29]   Inokubo Y, Hanada H, Ishizaka H, Fukushi T, Kamada T, Okumura K. Plasma levels of matrix metalloproteinase-9 and tissue inhibitor of metalloproteinase-1 are increased in the coronary circulation in patients with acute coronary syndrome. Am Heart J 2001; 141: 211-7.

[30]   Park JP, Lee BK, Shim JM, *et al.* Relationship between multiple plasma biomarkers and vulnerable plaque determined by virtual histology intravascular ultrasound. Circ J 2010; 74: 332-6.

[31]   Kadoglou NP, Gerasimidis T, Golemati S, Kapelouzou A, Karayannacos PE, Liapis CD. The relationship between serum levels of vascular calcification inhibitors and carotid plaque vulnerability. J Vasc Surg 2008; 47: 55-62.

[32]   Kadoglou NP, Sailer N, Moumtzouoglou A, Kapelouzou A, Gerasimidis T, Liapis CD. Aggressive lipid-lowering is more effective than moderate lipid-lowering treatment in carotid plaque stabilization. J Vasc Surg 2010; 51: 114-21.

[33]   Oei HH, van der Meer IM, Hofman A, *et al.* Lipoprotein-associated phospholipase A2 activity is associated with risk of coronary heart disease and ischemic stroke: the Rotterdam Study. Circulation 2005; 111: 570-5.

[34]   Zalewski A, Macphee C. Role of lipoprotein-associated phospholipase A2 in atherosclerosis: biology, epidemiology, and possible therapeutic target. Arterioscler Thromb Vasc Biol 2005; 25: 923-31.

[35]   Mallat Z, Lambeau G, Tedgui A. Lipoprotein-associated and secreted phospholipases A_2 in cardiovascular disease: roles as biological effectors and biomarkers. Circulation 2010; 122:2183-200.

[36]   Ehara S, Ueda M, Naruko T, *et al.* Elevated levels of oxidized low density lipoprotein show a positive relationship with the severity of acute coronary syndromes. Circulation 2001; 103: 1955-60.

[37]   Meisinger C, Baumert J, Khuseyinova N, Loewel H, Koenig W. Plasma oxidized low-density lipoprotein, a strong predictor for acute coronary heart disease events in apparently healthy, middle-aged men from the general population. Circulation 2005; 112: 651-7.

[38]   Fraley AE, Tsimikas S. Clinical applications of circulating oxidized low-density lipoprotein biomarkers in cardiovascular disease. Curr Opin Lipidol 2006; 17: 502-9.

[39]   Handberg A, Skjelland M, Michelsen AE, *et al.* Soluble CD36 in plasma is increased in patients with symptomatic atherosclerotic carotid plaques and is related to plaque instability. Stroke 2008; 39: 3092-5.

[40]   Spiel AO, Gilbert JC, Jilma B. von Willebrand factor in cardiovascular disease: focus on acute coronary syndromes. Circulation 2008; 117: 1449-59.

[41]   Páramo J, Beloqui O, Colina I, Diez J, Orbe J. Independent association of von Willebrand factor with surrogate markers of atherosclerosis in middle-aged asymptomatic subjects. J Thromb Haemost 2005; 3: 662-4.

[42]   Azuma RW, Kadowaki T, El-Saed A, *et al*. Associations of D-dimer and von Willebrand factor with atherosclerosis in Japanese and white men. Acta Cardiol 2010; 65: 449-56.
[43]   Cimmino G, Golino P, Badimon JJ. Pathophysiological role of blood-borne tissue factor: should the old paradigm be revisited? Intern Emerg Med 2011a; 6: 29-34.
[44]   Cimmino G, D'Amico C, Vaccaro V, D'Anna M, Golino P. The missing link between atherosclerosis, inflammation and thrombosis: is it tissue factor? Expert Rev Cardiovasc Ther 2011b; 9: 517-23.
[45]   Rautou PE, Vion AC, Amabile N, *et al*. Microparticles, vascular function, and atherothrombosis. Circ Res 2011; 109: 593-606.
[46]   Mallat Z, Hugel B, Ohan J, Lesèche G, Freyssinet JM, Tedgui A. Shed membrane microparticles with procoagulant potential in human atherosclerotic plaques: a role for apoptosis in plaque thrombogenicity. Circulation 1999; 99: 348-53.
[47]   Morel O, Toti F, Hugel B, *et al*. Procoagulant microparticles: disrupting the vascular homeostasis equation? Arterioscler Thromb Vasc Biol 2006; 26: 2594-604.
[48]   Wozniak SE, Gee LL, Wachtel MS, Frezza EE. Adipose tissue: the new endocrine organ? A review article. Dig Dis Sci 2009; 54: 1847-56.
[49]   Maia-Fernandes T, Roncon-Albuquerque R Jr, Leite-Moreira AF. Cardiovascular actions of adiponectin: pathophysiologic implications. Rev Port Cardiol 2008; 27: 1431-49.
[50]   Ekmekci H, Ekmekci OB. The role of adiponectin in atherosclerosis and thrombosis. Clin Appl Thromb Hemost 2006; 12: 163-8.
[51]   Barseghian A, Gawande D, Bajaj M. Adiponectin and vulnerable atherosclerotic plaques. J Am Coll Cardiol 2011; 57: 761-70.
[52]   Sawada T, Shite J, Shinke T, *et al*. Low plasma adiponectin levels are associated with presence of thin-cap fibroatheroma in men with stable coronary artery disease. Int J Cardiol 2010; 142: 250-6.
[53]   Gardener H, Sjoberg C, Crisby M, *et al*. Adiponectin and carotid intima-media thickness in the northern Manhattan study. Stroke 2012; 43: 1123-5.
[54]   Mohammadpour AH, Nazemian F, Moallem SA, Alamdaran SA, Asad-Abadi E, Shamsara J. Correlation between heat-shock protein 27 serum concentration and common carotid intima-media thickness in hemodialysis patients. Iran J Kidney Dis 2011; 5: 260-6.
[55]   Laufer EM, Mingels AM, Winkens MH, *et al*. The extent of coronary atherosclerosis is associated with increasing circulating levels of high sensitive cardiac troponin T. Arterioscler Thromb Vasc Biol. 2010; 30: 1269-75.
[56]   Kobayashi N, Hata N, Kume N, *et al*. Soluble lectin-like oxidized LDL receptor-1 and high-sensitivity troponin T as diagnostic biomarkers for acute coronary syndrome. Improved values with combination usage in emergency rooms. Circ J. 2011; 75: 2862-71.
[57]   Shah SH, de Lemos JA. Biomarkers and cardiovascular disease: determining causality and quantifying contribution to risk assessment. JAMA 2009; 302: 92-3.
[58]   Baldassarre D, De Jong A, Amato M, *et al*. Carotid intima-media thickness and markers of inflammation, endothelial damage and hemostasis. Ann Med 2008; 40: 21-44.
[59]   Ridker PM, Danielson E, Fonseca FA, Genest J, Gotto AM Jr, Kastelein JJ, Rosuvastatin to prevent vascular events in men and women with elevated C-reactive protein. N Engl J Med 2008; 359: 2195-207.
[60]   Ridker PM, Danielson E, Fonseca FA, *et al*. Reduction in C-reactive protein and LDL cholesterol and cardiovascular event rates after initiation of rosuvastatin: a prospective study of the JUPITER trial. Lancet 2009; 373: 1175-82.
[61]   Schroeder SA. Shattuck Lecture. We can do better--improving the health of the American people. N Engl J Med 2007; 357: 1221-8.
[62]   Elliott P, Chambers JC, Zhang W, *et al*. Genetic Loci associated with C-reactive protein levels and risk of coronary heart disease. JAMA 2009; 302: 37-48.
[63]   Pepys MB: CRP or not CRP? That is the question. Arterioscler Thromb Vasc Biol 2005; 25:1091- 4.
[64]   Melander O, Newton-Cheh C, Almgren P, *et al*., Novel and conventional biomarkers for prediction of incident cardiovascular events in the community. JAMA 2009; 302:49-57.
[65]   van Lammeren G, L Moll F, Borst GJ, de Kleijn DP, P M de Vries JP, Pasterkamp G. Atherosclerotic plaque biomarkers: beyond the horizon of the vulnerable plaque. Curr Cardiol Rev 2011; 7: 22-7.
[66]   Hazen SL. Myeloperoxidase and plaque vulnerability. Arterioscler Thromb Vasc Biol 2004; 24:1143-6.

[67] Baldus S, Heitzer T, Eiserich JP, *et al*. Myeloperoxidase enhances nitric oxide catabolism during myocardial ischemia and reperfusion. Free Radic Biol Med 2004; 37: 902-11.

[68] Ferrante G, Nakano M, Prati F, *et al*. High levels of systemic myeloperoxidase are associated with coronary plaque erosion in patients with acute coronary syndromes: a clinicopathological study. Circulation 2010; 122: 2505-13.

[69] Salonen I, Huttunen K, Hirvonen MR, *et al*. Serum myeloperoxidase is independent of the risk factors of atherosclerosis. Coron Artery Dis 2012

[70] Maier W, Altwegg LA, Corti R, *et al*. Inflammatory markers at the site of ruptured plaque in acute myocardial infarction: locally increased interleukin-6 and serum amyloid A but decreased C-reactive protein. Circulation 2005; 111: 1355-61.

[71] Koenig W, Khuseyinova N. Biomarkers of atherosclerotic plaque instability and rupture. Arterioscler Thromb Vasc Biol 2007; 27: 15-26.

[72] Mallat Z, Corbaz A, Scoazec A, *et al*. Expression of interleukin-18 in human atherosclerotic plaques and relation to plaque instability. Circulation 2001; 104: 1598-603.

[73] Aukrust P, Halvorsen B, Yndestad A, *et al*. Chemokines and cardiovascular risk. Arterioscler Thromb Vasc Biol 2008; 28: 1909-19.

[74] Rautou PE, Leroyer AS, Ramkhelawon B, *et al*. Microparticles from human atherosclerotic plaques promote endothelial ICAM-1-dependent monocyte adhesion and transendothelial migration. Circ Res 2011; 108: 335-43.

[75] Lievens D, Eijgelaar WJ, Biessen EA, Daemen MJ, Lutgens E. The multi-functionality of CD40L and its receptor CD40 in atherosclerosis. Thromb Haemost 2009; 102: 206-14.

[76] Schonbeck U, Libby P. CD40 signaling and plaque instability. Circ Res 2001; 89: 1092-1103.

[77] Lutgens E, Gorelik L, Daemen MJ, *et al*. Requirement for CD154 in the progression of atherosclerosis. Nat Med 1999; 5: 1313-1316.

[78] Lutgens E, Cleutjens KB, Heeneman S, *et al*. Both early and delayed anti-CD40L antibody treatment induces a stable plaque phenotype. Proc Natl Acad Sci USA 2000; 97: 7464-7469.

[79] Lutgens E, Daemen MJ. CD40-CD40L interactions in atherosclerosis. Trends Cardiovasc Med 2002; 12: 27-32.

[80] Mach F, Schönbeck U, Sukhova GK, *et al*. Reduction of atherosclerosis in mice by inhibition of CD40 signalling. Nature 1998; 394: 200-203.

[81] de Lemos JA, Zirlik A, Schonbeck U, *et al*. Associations between soluble CD40 ligand, atherosclerosis risk factors, and subclinical atherosclerosis: results from the Dallas Heart Study. Arterioscler Thromb Vasc Biol 2005; 25: 2192-6.

[82] Mason DP, Kenagy RD, Hasenstab D, *et al*. Matrix metalloproteinase-9 overexpression enhances vascular smooth muscle cell migration and alters remodeling in the injured rat carotid artery. Circ Res 1999; 85: 1179-85.

[83] Momiyama Y, Ohmori R, Tanaka N, *et al*. High plasma levels of matrix metalloproteinase-8 in patients with unstable angina. Atherosclerosis 2010; 209: 206-10.

[84] Djurić T, Zivković M, Stanković A, *et al*. Plasma levels of matrix metalloproteinase-8 in patients with carotid atherosclerosis. J Clin Lab Anal 2010; 24: 246-51.

[85] Jones GT, Tarr GP, Phillips LV, Wilkins GT, van Rij AM, Williams MJ. Active matrix metalloproteinases 3 and 9 are independently associated with coronary artery in-stent restenosis. Atherosclerosis 2009; 207: 603-7.

[86] Deguchi JO, Aikawa M, Tung CH, *et al*. Inflammation in atherosclerosis: visualizing matrix metalloproteinase action in macrophages in vivo. Circulation 2006; 114: 55-62.

[87] Golledge J, McCann M, Mangan S, Lam A, Karan M. Osteoprotegerin and osteopontin are expressed at high concentrations within symptomatic carotid atherosclerosis. Stroke 2004; 35: 1636-41.

[88] Jenny NS. Lipoprotein-associated phospholipase A2: novel biomarker and causal mediator of atherosclerosis? Arterioscler Thromb Vasc Biol 2006; 26: 2417-8.

[89] Kolodgie FD, Burke AP, Skorija KS, *et al*. Lipoprotein-associated phospholipase A2 protein expression in the natural progression of human coronary atherosclerosis. Arterioscler Thromb Vasc Biol 2006; 26: 2523-9.

[90] Serruys PW, García-García HM, Buszman P, *et al*. Effects of the direct lipoprotein-associated phospholipase A(2) inhibitor darapladib on human coronary atherosclerotic plaque. Circulation 2008; 118: 1172-82.

[91]   Ali M, Madjid M. Lipoprotein-associated phospholipase A2: a cardiovascular risk predictor and a potential therapeutic target. Future Cardiol 2009; 5: 159-73.

[92]   Yang H, Mohamed AS, Zhou SH. Oxidized low density lipoprotein, stem cells, and atherosclerosis. Lipids Health Dis 2012; 11: 85.

[93]   Imazu M, Ono K, Tadehara F, *et al.* Plasma levels of oxidized low density lipoprotein are associated with stable angina pectoris and modalities of acute coronary syndrome. Int Heart J 2008, 49: 515-24.

[94]   Sigala F, Kotsinas A, Savari P, *et al.* Oxidized LDL in human carotid plaques is related to symptomatic carotid disease and lesion instability. J Vasc Surg 2010; 52: 704-13.

[95]   Handberg A, Højlund K, Gastaldelli A, *et al.* Plasma sCD36 is associated with markers of atherosclerosis, insulin resistance and fatty liver in a nondiabetic healthy population. J Intern Med 2012; 271: 294-304.

[96]   Nakagawa-Toyama Y, Yamashita S, Miyagawa J, *et al.* Localization of CD36 and scavenger receptor class A in human coronary arteries--a possible difference in the contribution of both receptors to plaque formation. Atherosclerosis 2001; 156: 297-305.

[97]   van der Wal AC, Li X, de Boer OJ. Tissue factor expression in the morphologic spectrum of vulnerable atherosclerotic plaques. Semin Thromb Hemost 2006; 32: 40-7.

[98]   Cimmino G, Conte S, Morello A, D'Elia S, Marchese V, Golino P. The complex puzzle underlying the pathophysiology of acute coronary syndromes: from molecular basis to clinical manifestations. Expert Rev Cardiovasc Ther 2012; 10: 1533-43.

[99]   Glaudemans AW, Slart RH, Bozzao A, *et al.* Molecular imaging in atherosclerosis. Eur J Nucl Med Mol Imaging 2010; 37: 2381-97.

[100]   ten Kate GL, Sijbrands EJ, Valkema R, *et al.* Molecular imaging of inflammation and intraplaque vasa vasorum: a step forward to identification of vulnerable plaques? J Nucl Cardiol 2010; 17: 897-912.

[101]   Sadeghi MM, Glover DK, Lanza GM, Fayad ZA, Johnson LL. Imaging atherosclerosis and vulnerable plaque. J Nucl Med 2010; 51 S1: 51S-65S.

[102]   Owen DR, Lindsay AC, Choudhury RP, Fayad ZA. Imaging of atherosclerosis. Annu Rev Med 2011; 62: 25-40.

[103]   Soloperto G, Casciaro S. Progress in atherosclerotic plaque imaging. World J Radiol 2012; 4: 353-71.

[104]   Temma T, Saji H. Radiolabelled probes for imaging of atherosclerotic plaques. Am J Nucl Med Mol Imaging 2012; 2: 432-47.

[105]   Osborn EA, Jaffer FA. Imaging atherosclerosis and risk of plaque rupture. Curr Atheroscler Rep 2013; 15: 359.

[106]   Saba L, Anzidei M, Marincola BC, *et al.* Imaging of the Carotid Artery Vulnerable Plaque. Cardiovasc Intervent Radiol 2013.

[107]   Fleg JL, Stone GW, Fayad ZA, *et al.* Detection of high-risk atherosclerotic plaque: report of the NHLBI Working Group on current status and future directions. JACC Cardiovasc Imaging. 2012; 5 :941-55.

[108]   Cocker MS, Mc Ardle B, Spence JD, *et al.* Imaging atherosclerosis with hybrid [(18)F]fluorodeoxyglucose positron emission tomography/computed tomography imaging: what Leonardo da Vinci could not see. J Nucl Cardiol. 2012; 19: 1211-25.

22

Tissue Factor Structure and Coagulation

Jolanta Krudysz-Amblo, Kenneth G. Mann and Saulius Butenas[*]

University of Vermont, Department of Biochemistry, Burlington, Vermont, USA

Abstract: This chapter describes the structure-function relationship of tissue factor (TF) also known as coagulation factor III, tissue thromboplastin, and CD142. Tissue factor is a procoagulant transmembrane glycoprotein and is essential to life. This single chain protein belongs to a Cytokine Receptor Superfamily (CRS) with a Fibronectin Type III topology. Proteins of the CRS group are transmembrane receptor proteins and fibronectins have been implicated in numerous functions such as blood clotting, wound healing, metastasis, cell signaling and embryogenesis. Tissue factor initiates the extrinsic pathway of blood coagulation leading to thrombin generation and clot formation. In addition to its primary role in coagulation, TF has also been an important player in many biological processes. Tissue factor is expressed by cells of arteriosclerotic lesions associated with plaque rupture in the vasculature. In addition, calcium- and phosphorylation-dependent regulation of TF makes it an important molecule in signal transduction and cell-to-cell interactions in the vasculature. In oncology, TF has been described as a marker of cancer development and a prometastatic molecule. The numerous functions of TF contribute to its importance in human biology. Although presently it is most prominently known for its role in coagulation, evolutionary sequence homologies and similar structural topologies with fibronectins of the CRS proteins place TF in a much wider spectrum of functions.

Keywords: Tissue factor, isolation, biochemical characterization, structure, posttranslational modifications, carbohydrates, phosphorylation, cysteines and disulfides, complex with factor VIIa, activity, extrinsic factor Xase, mass-spectrometry.

INTRODUCTION

Acute coronary syndromes (ACS) are a major cause of death in developed countries. The leading cause of ACS is an atherosclerotic plaque disruption and subsequent thrombosis. In its turn, atherosclerotic plaque development is closely related to inflammatory processes and enhanced procoagulant activity [1]. Plaque growth is up-regulated by pro-inflammatory cytokines, which are increased in

---

*Corresponding author Saulius Butenas: University of Vermont, Department of Biochemistry, Burlington, Vermont, USA; Tel: +1-802-656-0350; Fax: +1-802-656-2256; E-mail: sbutenas@uvm.edu.

ACS patients [2] and can also stimulate tissue factor (TF) expression [3]. As a consequence, increased levels of circulating TF are observed in ACS patients [4-9]. With TF being a key initiator of blood coagulation *in vivo*, it is not surprising that elevated levels of this protein lead to a prothrombotic phenotype. In addition to TF, several other coagulation proteins, such as factor VII, factor VIII and prothrombin [10-13], are elevated in ACS patients. A further increase in the thrombotic risk could be caused by the presence of activated factor XIa circulating in ACS patient blood [4]. In contrast to coagulation proteins, a decrease in the concentration of several coagulation inhibitors, such as antithrombin-III, protein C and protein S, are also observed in subjects with ACS [14-17]. The data related to the concentration of other key coagulation inhibitor, tissue factor pathway inhibitor, are somewhat controversial. It has been suggested in the majority of publications that concentration of this inhibitor is elevated in ACS subjects [5, 11, 18, 19], such increase was not able to compensate for elevated TF concentrations [5, 6]. As a result of interplay between the concentrations of procoagulants and coagulation inhibitors, an increase in thrombin generation and clot formation are observed in blood and plasma of patients [11, 20-22]. Moreover, thrombotic complications could be further propagated by an impaired fibrinolytic system due to an elevated concentration of plasminogen activator inhibitor-1 and an imbalance between this inhibitor and a plasminogen activator [6, 23, 24]. Due to the role TF plays in ACS, we are going to discuss some well-established facts related to TF and some controversial observations addressing TF structure-function relationships.

TF is a 263 amino acid glycoprotein containing three domains: the extracellular domain (residues 1-219), the transmembrane domain (residues 220-242) and the cytoplasmic domain (residues 243-263) [25]. Fig. **1** demonstrates the schematic representation of the three domains of TF.

The extracellular domain binds the zymogen/enzyme factor (F)VII/FVIIa and the molecular substrates FIX and FX. The transmembrane domain serves as an anchor to the cell membrane, whereas the cytoplasmic domain has been suggested to play a role in signal transduction. Tissue factor is essential to life and human TF deficiency has yet to be identified. Mice lacking TF die during embryonic development [26]. Tissue factor is an integral membrane glycoprotein which upon stimulus is exposed on cellular surfaces to circulating blood FVIIa. Fig. **2** demonstrates the assembly of the extrinsic FXase, intrinsic FXase and prothrombinase complexes. The TF-FVIIa complex assembly accelerates the

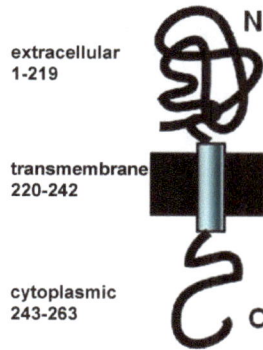

Figure 1: Presentation of TF protein as a single chain transmembrane glycoprotein. The extracellular N-terminal region consists of residues 1-219, transmembrane domain of residues 220-242 and cytoplasmic domain of residues 243-263.

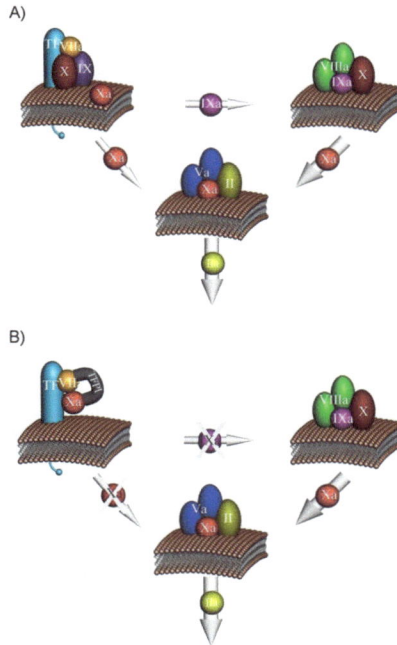

Figure 2: Complex formation of the extrinsic factor FXase composed of TF-FVIIa, intrinsic FXase composed of FVIIIa-FIXa and prothrombinase composed of FVa-FXa. The extrinsic FXase complex, TF-FVIIa, activates FIX to FIXa and FX to FXa. The latter converts prothrombin to thrombin. FV and FVIII are in turn activated by thrombin produced and form the prothrombinase and intrinsic FXase complexes, respectively. (**A**) FXa is generated 50-fold more efficiently by the intrinsic FXase (thick arrow) than by the extrinsic FXase. (**B**) The tissue factor pathway inhibitor (TFPI) inhibits the TF-FVIIa-FXa complex and blocks the formation of FIXa and FXa by the extrinsic FXase catalyst. (Used with permission from: Mann KG. Dynamics in Hemostasis. Haematologic Technologies 2002).

generation of activated FX (FXa) by 7 orders of magnitude [27]. The serine proteases, activated FIX (FIXa) and FXa, form the intrinsic FXase with FVIIIa and the prothrombinase complex with FVa, respectively, which lead to robust thrombin generation and subsequently to clot formation [28, 29]. The interaction of TF with FVIIa is calcium dependent and the proteolysis of both FIX and FX by the complex is membrane dependent [30, 31].

The cascade of enzymatic events resulting in the formation of a fibrin matrix and its dissolution is the main defense of the vascular system. The complex system of blood coagulation and its regulation consists of numerous enzymes, factors and cofactors and is responsible in maintaining the haemostatic balance between thrombosis and hemorrhage [32]. Upon damage or injury to the vasculature, the circulating and non-circulating proteins enter a process of protein interactions required for procoagulant events leading to thrombin generation. Clot formation and its subsequent fibrinolysis is an equilibrium that must be maintained to prevent bleeding or excessive clot formation thus compromising the entire system [33]. Regulation of blood coagulation involves initiation by the extrinsic pathway and amplification by the intrinsic pathway (Fig. **2**). The extrinsic pathway consists of the complex formed by the transmembrane receptor TF and circulating plasma FVII/FVIIa. This high affinity extrinsic FXase complex leads to the activation of serine proteases, FIX and FX, resulting in the conversion of fibrinogen to fibrin and formation of a stable clot [34]. The intrinsic pathway involves the hemophilia factors VIII and IX [35]. In hemostasis, upon injury, circulating blood components are exposed to subendothelial vessel wall expressing TF and therefore initiating blood clotting. In thrombosis, pathologic conditions lead to the expression of TF on cells, primarily on monocytes and possibly on endothelial. The role of TF in thrombosis and hemorrhage has been investigated and described [32].

HISTORY

The fascination with the clotting of blood dates back to the times of Aristotle and Plato [36, 37]. Investigations of coagulation during the 18th and 19th centuries, although informative, occurred without the complete understanding of the underlying molecular mechanisms [38]. The importance of tissue extracts, especially of brain extracts, in activation or hastening of blood coagulation was reported as early as 1869 by Carpenter in "Principles of human physiology" and said to be known since 1834 [39]. The chemical nature of the substance contained in the tissue extracts was preliminarily studied by Wooldridge as early as 1883. It was also at that time that it was identified as a phospholipin-protein complex [40]. Further recognition of the tissue based trigger of blood coagulation, called "zymoplastic substance" by Schmidt, proved to be an important stepping stone in elucidating the phenomena of blood clotting [38]. The role of the coagulation trigger, then named thromboplastin, as the major player in blood coagulation was assigned by Loeb and Morawitz in the early 1900's [41]. By the early 20th century a preliminary pathway of coagulation had been developed and better molecular techniques allowed for the identification and purification of coagulation proteins. Tissue factor or thromboplastin was found to be expressed in most animal tissues and it was discovered to be released upon wound production [42, 43].

By 1929 the classical theory of blood coagulation was postulated to take place in two phases. Phase one consisted of the conversion of prothrombin, in the presence of calcium and thromboplastin, to thrombin. Phase two required the thrombin component to form fibrin from fibrinogen. The factor which required calcium ions to convert prothrombin to thrombin was identified by various names such as thromboplastin, thrombokinase, thrombozyme, cytozyme, today known as TF. The thermostable factor or clotting activator was also identified as a phosphotide, belonging to the cephalin group of proteins [38]. It was believed for some time that the active factor was cephalin alone [42]. However, in due course the active substance was discovered to consist of two components, a lipid component and a protein component [39]. This finding was solely supported by the early work of Wooldridge who recognized the material to be a phospholipin-protein complex [40]. Further investigations over the next few decades led to the elucidation of the coagulation cascade and its players. The coagulation trigger, now commonly known as TF, has proved to be an important element in many biological processes. Its role in hemostasis, thrombosis, cancer, inflammation, angiogenesis and embryogenesis has been substantiated [44]. This review chapter covers the few major aspects of TF structure and function.

ISOLATION

The interest in the substance, or TF, responsible for the initiation of blood coagulation led to the intensive design of purification techniques. Early extraction of testes, thymus, and lymph nodes by Wooldridge showed that strong acidification with acetic acid precipitated the active material. Extraction of the precipitate with alcohol or ether destroyed its clotting activity. The instantaneous toxicity of the substance, when injected into animals, was initially reported by Wooldridge [40]. A few other studies following the work of Wooldridge also described the factor in tissue extracts as toxic since it produced death in animals upon injection [39].

Various methods for the isolation of the clotting factor were investigated profoundly by Mills [39]. Lung tissue of dogs, rabbits and cattle was used for the extraction of the substance, since it was observed to contain more of the active material than other tissues. Ammonium sulfate or magnesium sulfate, mercury chloride, sulfosalicylic acid and sulfuric acid were used as precipitants of the active material. Mills established the isoelectric point to be between pH 5 and pH 6 [39]. An improved procedure for the isolation of the protein component and phospholipid component from beef lung, using the method of fractional salt precipitation, was developed. Isolated phospholipids showed negligible activity in contrast to thromboplastin. The precipitated protein alone also showed no activity [45].

Fractional ultracentrifugation as a means of isolation of the thromboplastin component was employed by Chargaff *et al.*, [46]. It was observed that this method leads to very active and homogenous preparations with respect to electrophoretic mobility and sedimentation velocity, however in very small lots. The effect on the disintegration of the protein from the phospholipid component by the use of denaturants such as guanidine and sodium deoxycholate was initially observed by Chargaff [43]. Partially purified protein was successfully obtained in the 1970s with preliminary analysis on sodium dodecyl sulfate polyacrylamide gel electrophoresis (SDS-PAGE) [47, 48]. Further improvements allowed for more precise quantitation and characterization of the protein component [49, 50]. It was noted at the time that the purified protein had a marked tendency to aggregate at all stages of the purification procedure. The inclusion of detergents throughout the isolation process prevented the formation of aggregates [50]. By the early 1980s a method for isolation of TF was developed using Triton-X100, an anionic detergent [51-53]. The employment of Triton-X100 in isolation and affinity purification on FVII-coupled resin resulted in purity comparable to that obtained by the method of affinity by antibody (Ab) chromatography.

BIOCHEMICAL CHARACTERIZATION

Early studies on the chemical composition and the electrophoretic properties of the thromboplastic protein from bovine lungs was carried out by Cohen and coworkers [54, 55]. The lipoprotein was obtained by isoelectric point precipitation and shown to contain not only lipids but steroids, steroid esters, and natural glycerides. Subsequently, the physical data by sedimentation in an ultracentrifuge was obtained by Chargaff *et al.*, [46]. The isolation of the human protein *via* a repeated preparative polyacrylamide gel electrophoresis method permitted the assessment of the approximate molecular weight to be 52 kilodaltons (kDa) [48, 56]. Bjorklid and co-investigators further characterized the thromboplastin protein with respect to the amino acid, lipid and carbohydrate content [50]. The obtained amino acid composition allowed for the approximation of the molecular weight to 52 kDa. It became evident that the high hydrophobic amino acid content of 42%, presumably clustered on the molecule, attributed to the tendency of the protein to aggregate in detergent-free solution. This suggested that the cluster of hydrophobic amino acids is sufficient to keep the protein embedded in a cellular membrane [50].

The first use of Triton-X100 in conjunction with affinity column chromatography allowed for a relatively homogenous preparation. Analysis by SDS-PAGE revealed a 43 kDa molecule, which differed from that found by Bjorklid and coworkers with a molecular weight of 52 kDa. The discrepancy was attributed to the difference in species or the method of purification [51]. Guha *et al.*, presented evidence that TF purified to homogeneity by TritonX-100 extraction exhibits an apparent molecular weight of 46 kDa by SDS-PAGE and retains its activity in detergent micelles, although to a lesser extent than when reconstituted in lipids [53]. The molecular weight of 46 kDa has been used throughout literature as the molecular weight of the natural protein. More recently the use of mass spectrometry allowed for a more direct measurement of the molecular weight of 36 kDa than that achievable by SDS-PAGE [57].

GENE STRUCTURE, ORGANIZATION AND PRIMARY SEQUENCE

The TF gene was found to be located on chromosome 1p21-22 spanning approximately 12.4 kilobases (kb). The amino acid sequence has been determined from the cloned 2.3 kb cDNA, containing 263 residues in the mature protein (Fig. **1**) after the cleavage of a 32 residue leader sequence [25, 58-61]. The coding sequence is made up of six exons. Exon one corresponds to the propetide and the translation initiation sites. Exons two to five contain sites for the translation of the extracellular domain of the molecule consisting of 219 residues. Exon six constitutes the 23 residue transmembrane region and the 21 residue cytoplasmic domain [62]. Comparison of human TF cDNA with that of bovine, murine, rat and rabbit shows a high degree of sequence conservation within a range of 50 to 70 percent [63-66]. The 5' untranslated region of TF gene includes the promoter region with consensus sequences from human, murine, and porcine species for binding of transcription factors Sp1, EGR1, AP-1, AP-2, and NF-κB, and two CACCC sites [67-72].

The analysis of the TF sequence revealed a distant homology to the cytokine receptor superfamily [73]. The primary sequence, as well as structural homology, places TF with a group of receptors such as the human growth hormone receptor, prolactin, erythropoietin receptor, the interferon-γ receptor, CD2, and CD4 [74-79]. The solution of the three dimensional structure of the extracellular region of these proteins and that of TF (Figs. **3** and **4**) shows a domain formed by two immunoglobulin like modules. The amino terminus (N-terminus) of TF consists of residues 1-219, is extracellular and is composed of two domains joined at an angle of 125 degrees. The N-terminus of the molecule is located on the outside of the cell [79]. The cleft formed at the interface between the two immunoglobulin-like modules was predicted to serve as the ligand binding site. Studies demonstrate that TF is expressed early on in human development prior to the formation of circulation system and prior to the detectable expression of FVII, possibly assigning a secondary role to that in coagulation and consistent with the grouping of TF as a receptor. It was therefore suggested that other roles, such as signaling, and other ligands might exist for TF outside of coagulation, possibly in the early development of the central nervous system and the cardiovascular system [80, 81].

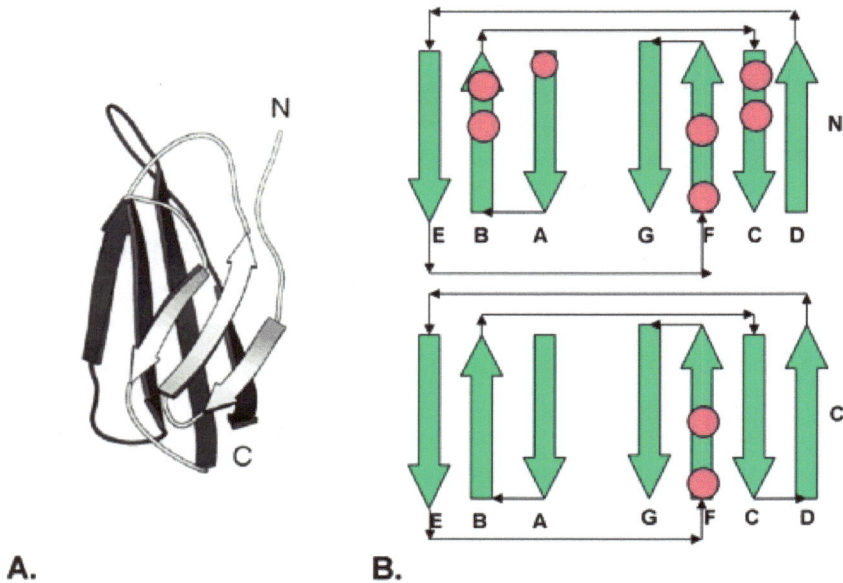

A.   **B.**

Figure 3: (A) Schematic presentation of fibronectin III type toplogy consisting of seven antiparallel beta-sheets (B) Presentation of fibronectin III type N- and C-domains showing connectivity of the antiparallel beta sheets and their arrangement into a sandwich Greek key motif. The N- and C-domains constitute the extracellular domain of fibronectin III type proteins including TF. (This Figure was originally published in: Butenas S. Tissue factor structure and function. Scientifica 2012; 2012:964862.).

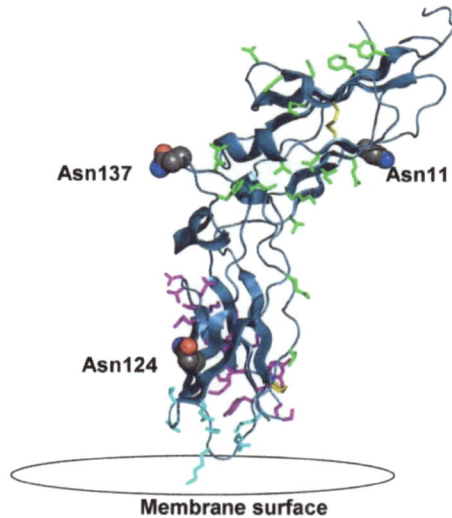

Figure 4: The extracellular domain (residues 1-219) of human TF on a modeled lipid membrane. Highlighted in red are three sites of N-linked glycosylation at Asn11, Asn124 and Asn137. Highlighted in green are residues important for TF interaction with FVIIa, in magenta are residues important for the interaction with FX and in aqua are the residues important for TF interaction with the membrane. Shown in yellow are the two disulfide bridges of TF at positions Cys49-Cys57 and Cys186-Cys209. [This Figure was originally published in: Krudysz-Amblo *et al.*, Differences in the fractional abundances of carbohydrates of natural and recombinant human tissue factor. Biochim Biophys Acta 2011; 1810: 398-405 (see reference 183)].

MEMBER OF THE CYTOKINE RECEPTOR SUPERFAMILY

Tissue factor, a member of the class 2 cytokine receptor superfamily (CRF) and Fibronectin type III (FNIII) family is found/expressed on fibroblasts, smooth muscle cells, keratinocytes, monocytes and endothelial cells and is upregulated by exposure to bacterial endotoxins, proinflammatory molecules and pathological conditions [34]. The cytokine receptor superfamily comprises a diverse group of proteins with significantly homologous binding domains. The binding domains constitute a ~200 residue long segment with conserved regions of beta-strands. The structural analysis of the distinctive binding domain shows a homology in sequence and structure topology. Fig. **3** presents the characteristic antiparallel beta-sandwich fold with a Greek key motif, a domain with a strong implication of evolutionary emergence of a class of regulatory receptor molecules. These motifs are found in the extracellular domains of a subgroup of receptor family proteins such as interferon-α/β, γ receptors and TF. The motif is also linked to the immunoglobulin superfamily with the analogous antiparallel β-sandwich topology [73, 82].

Fibronectins are glycoproteins involved in numerous important cellular processes such as blood clotting, tissue repair, wound healing, cell migration, cell adhesion, tumor metastasis, cell differentiation and embryogenesis. The wide spectrum of activities of the molecules in signaling and binding necessitates its interaction with various ligands including collagen, DNA, heparin, actins, fibrin and receptors on cell surfaces [73, 83].

In addition, TF is characterized as a member of the cytokine/hematopoietic growth factor receptor family based on its distant sequence similarities, topology and a receptor like function. Proteins belonging to this family are cell-surface molecules with a single transmembrane domain and a cytoplasmic domain with structural diversity. The unique characteristic of this family is a distinct disulfide bond in the extracellular domain further dividing the group into class 1 receptors including human growth hormone receptor, interleukin receptors, and hematopoietin growth factor receptors and class 2 receptors including TF, interferon receptors, and IL-10 receptor [84].

DISTRIBUTION

By the mid-1900s Astrup *et al.*, examined the distribution of TF in the human body observing high levels of activity in the brain, lungs and kidney [85]. The development and use of polyclonal and then monoclonal antibodies allowed for the localization of TF to vascular adventitia, organ capsules, epithelium of skin, and mucosa [86-89]. Faulk and coworkers identified the TF presenting cells in human placenta by immunohistologic studies [87]. Observations revealed that TF is found on some macrophages, most fibroblast-like cells, occasionally in perivascular cells and endothelium. Chorionic villi showed positive staining for TF but only on the sections presenting histological evidence of chronic inflammation [87]. Furthermore, Lockwood *et al.*, demonstrated that decidualization of endometrial stromal cells is accompanied by a significant increase in the expression of TF. The presence of TF in decidualized cells suggests a mechanism by which hemorrhage is evaded during trophoblast invasion of the endometrial vasculature [89].

Tissue factor is constitutively expressed by certain cells associated with the vessel wall including vascular smooth muscle cells, adventitial fibroblasts and pericytes [90, 91]. High levels are found specifically in the astrocytes of brain tissue, epithelial cells of the lung and cardiomyocytes in the heart [92]. The expression of TF by endothelium is somewhat controversial. Endothelial cells in the vessel are crucial for vascular hemostasis. Endothelial TF expression has been suggested in individuals with sickle cell disease, tumors, leukemia patients, individuals with atherosclerosis and inflammatory bowel disease [93-97]. Whether healthy endothelium expresses TF is still debatable. It has been demonstrated that TF expression on cultured endothelial cells could be induced [98]. The expression of both the full-length form as well as a soluble form, more commonly called alternatively spliced TF, has been described [99, 100]. Although the procoagulant contribution of the two forms seems to be debatable, the inductive factors for their expression are believed to be inflammatory cytokines, specifically tumor-necrosis-factor-α (TNF-α) and interleukin-6 (IL-6) [99, 101]. On the contrary, reports of other investigators conclude that TF is not detectable in the endothelium [102, 103].

Tissue factor expression on circulating cells has been of great interest. Induction of circulating monocytes with lipopolysaccharides (LPS) has been shown to induce TF expression *in vitro* and *in vivo* [104, 105]. Stimulation of monocytes through inflammatory pathways has also been described [106]. TF expression on neutrophils has also been somewhat debatable. If detected, expression is usually associated with disease and endotoxemia [107]. Circulating microparticles containing TF, generated by endothelial cells, leukocytes and vascular smooth muscle cells, have been described. Microparticles are small anucleoid cell membrane fragments shed from cells including platelets, monocytes, erythrocytes, leukocytes, and endothelial cells [108-111]. They are believed to exist in healthy individuals but increase in number due to pathological conditions [112]. The small membrane fragments contribute to thrombosis, especially in patients with cardiovascular disease, cancer, sickle cell disease, diabetes and endotoxemia [113-116]. They facilitate cellular interactions through cell signaling pathways and upon injury or stimulus accumulate in a clot and contribute to thrombus formation [117]. Aharon and coworkers [118] demonstrated that microparticles, originating from monocytes, attach to endothelial cells and stimulate their dysfunction and thrombogenicity.

Imposed damage to the endothelium by activated monocytes has been associated with increased microparticle production and therefore TF-dependent procoagulant activity [119]. It has been reported that TF concentration on microparticles is higher than that of the parent cell. This may be attributed to the increased concentration of phosphotidylserine on the outer leaflet of the membrane and "de-encryption" of TF [120]. It has been suggested that the parent cell determines the fate of the microparticle, *i.e.* monocyte microparticles induce von Willebrand factor expression on endothelial cells and leukocyte microparticles transfer TF to platelets [121, 122]. Endothelial cell microparticles possess markers expressed upon stimulation on mature cells [123]. Following cytokine stimulation, some microparticles gain the ability to initiate coagulation through increased expression of TF [124].

The existence of TF on platelets has been controversial and still an unresolved phenomena. The sources of TF in platelets have been described to include de-novo synthesis and storage in α-granules as well as absorption of microparticle-TF. Early studies by Zillmann *et al.*, suggested that platelets isolated from stimulated blood contain TF that is functional [125]. Muller *et al.*, claimed the presence of TF in α-granules of resting platelets [126]. Panes *et al.*, believed that platelets synthesize TF in response to activation [127]. Other studies suggested the presence of TF mRNA in platelets [128, 129]. The observed presence of TF in platelets would change the scheme of the coagulation pathway implicating that TF may contribute not only to the initiation phase but also to the amplification phase of coagulation. These observations have been challenged. Butenas *et al.*, observed no detectable activity or antigen in inactive and ionophore stimulated platelets [130]. Similarly, Osterud failed to detect any TF activity in collagen stimulated platelets [131]. Bouchard and coworkers also observed that human platelets stimulated with PAR-1 and PAR-4 agonist peptides do not express TF [132].

The presence of a non-bound form of alternatively spliced soluble TF in blood has also been noted, however once again with conflicting messages. The source and the functional role in coagulation, if any, have baffled many investigators [133-136]. Tissue factor in blood may also be detected as a form of a degradation product and not necessarily as an alternatively spliced form [130]. Reported concentrations of up to 10 nM of functional protein in blood exceed the sub(picomal) concentrations required to initiate a clot within a few minutes [137]. Studies from our laboratory and others report that if TF circulates in whole blood, the concentrations of it do not exceed 20 fM [130, 138]. Using our assays, we report that TF antigen concentrations in acute coronary syndrome patient plasmas reach only picomolar levels with no more than 0.4 pM of functional protein in the majority of patient samples [130]. The observed discrepancies in circulating TF concentrations may be attributed to the shortcomings and poor validation of commercially-available assays used by various laboratories [4, 139, 140]. In conclusion, it has been accepted, in general, that blood-borne TF does not play significant (if any) role in blood coagulation.

ROLE IN BLOOD COAGULATION

Membrane-Dependent Activity

The early notion that phospholipids are essential for the clotting activity of the protein substance from tissue extracts stemmed from the studies of Wooldridge [40]. Digestion with pepsin-HCl produced a precipitate of the phospholipin component with little protein content. Clotting was not efficient with either the precipitate or the solution of the digest, which suggested that the substance was a protein-phospholipin complex. It also suggested that the phopsholipin was essential for the clotting activity of the protein component [39]. Mills was the pioneer in the absolute determination that both the protein and the phospholipin component are essential for the activity of the tissue extract. By recombining the separated inactive protein and phospholipin components Mills confirmed that the activity was restored upon the protein-phospholipin complex formation. It was also noted that the concentration of phospholipid is very important for the activity of the protein component [54, 141, 142].

The composition of the lipid fraction of thromboplastin was initially described by Cohen *et al.*, [54] and Chargaff *et al.*, [143]. The reported tentative lipid composition of bovine lung thromboplastin consisted of 19% cholesterol, 63% phospholipids (26% lecithin, 25% cephalin, 12% sphingomyelin) and 18% fat. Other investigators observed that reconstitution of a single phospholipid–protein mixtures restored partial activity when phosphatidylethanolamine and to a lesser extent phosphatidylcholine were used, whereas phosphotidylserine and phosphotidylinositol were ineffective [142, 144, 145]. Subsequent studies performed by Bjorklid *et al.*, [50] demonstrated a lipid composition similar to that reported by Chargaff and coworkers. The lipid content was reported to consist of 34-43% phosphatidylcholine, 12-23% cholesterol plus free fatty acids, 13-22% phosphatidylethanolamine, 5-16% lysophosphatidylcholine, 7-9% sphingomyelin, 6-7% phosphatidylserine, and traces of phosphatidylinositol. Nemerson has shown that both active and inactive lipids were bound equally to TF, speculating that the activity is not a function of binding but the chemical nature of the bound lipid [146].

In contrast to Nemerson, Pitlick, Liu, Bjorklid and their coworkers showed that phosphotidylserine was more effective than phosphotidylcholine in restoring partial activity of TF [50, 142, 144, 145]. All groups agreed that binary phospholipid systems were much more effective and ternary systems exceedingly effective in restoring full procoagulant activity of TF. Eventually, phosphatidylserine was assigned as having an essential role in the enhancement of TF activity. Its introduction into a phosphotidylcholine and phosphotidylethanolamine mixture increased the activity of the thromboplastin protein by 100-fold [50]. Bull *et al.*, closely examined the importance of phosphatidylserine by indicating that the negative charge, of the lipid facilitates at physiological pH FX and FII (prothrombin) binding to the membrane through

Ca^{++} bridges [147]. Bach *et al.*, suggested that phosphatidylserine may be the component in a signal transduction pathway by which TF "decryption" occurs, resulting in an increased procoagulant activity when cells undergo stimulation by calmodulin-mediated events [120].

In summary, many investigators have stressed the important role of the phospholipid component and its charge in the activity of blood coagulation proteins. The discrepancies arise in the specific activity of each phospholipid, specifically their contribution to the activity of TF. By using biological membranes, Marcus and coworkers have shown that lipoproteins embedded in a form of a platelet membrane are more active than lipoproteins reconstituted in lipid micelles [148]. Similar results were observed by Butenas and coworkers where monocyte cell surface TF is more than 100-fold more active than purified, relipidated monocyte TF [149]. The results of the study indicate that a positive correlation exists between TF activity and TF antigen of the monocytic cell, contradictory to the "encryption" theory. The authors suggest that cell membrane components, including specific lipids or an unidentified receptor, attribute to the enhanced activity.

Complex Formation with FVIIa

By the early 1960s it was shown that FVII in combination with tissue extracts hastens blood coagulation by activating FX. It was suggested that FVII has an enzymatic activity [150-153]. Nemerson established that TF interacts with FVII forming an intermediate which is responsible for FX activation. The interaction between TF and FX was postulated to be lipid and Ca^{++} dependent, whereas the connectivity between TF and FVII remained obscure [153]. The assignment of FX as a substrate of TF-FVII and the involvement of the complex in the extrinsic pathway of coagulation was then reported by Silverberg *et al.*, [154]. The recognition of TF as an obligatory cofactor for "FVII enzyme" was therefore established. At the same time Osterud and coworkers reported the involvement of TF and FVII in the classical intrinsic pathway by the ability of the complex to activate FIX [155].

The mechanism of the TF pathway and of FVII proteolysis was extensively studied by Nemerson [156]. The direct activation of FX by the TF–FVIIa complex was established by Jesty [157]. The authors suggested a dual role for FVII in which FVII circulates as a low activity species zymogen but only exhibits its maximum proteolytic activity when in complex with TF. The key evidence that FVII is a zymogen and FVIIa is the enzyme stemmed from the studies of Lawson and coworkers [158]. Factor VII was eventually recognized as an inert zymogen which in complex with TF cannot activate measurable amounts of FX. However the rapid conversion or activation of TF bound FVII and formation of the TF-VIIa complex serves as a potent initiator of the TF dependent coagulation pathway [159]. Studies concluded that vessel wall injury attracts circulating FVII/FVIIa to bind TF expressed on cells in the vessel, leading to the formation of TF-FVIIa complex. The trace amount of FXa generated activates FVII to FVIIa only in the TF–FVII complex which in turn amplifies the rapid conversion of FX to FXa. The interplay between TF, FVII, FVIIa and FX is a key control point for the profound effect in the initiation of the extrinsic pathway of blood coagulation [159].

Factor VIIa possesses extremely low activity when free in circulation or with phospholipid alone in the absence of its cofactor TF. The extracellular domain of TF is involved in protein–protein interactions with the single-chain FVII or the two-chain FVIIa. Tissue factor is required for the catalytic enhancement of FVIIa and the subsequent substrate cleavage by its catalytic domain. The activity of the complex is optimal when TF is expressed on a surface of a cell or on a phospholipid membrane. The high affinity binding of TF for FVII or FVIIa requires between 2–5 mM of Ca^{++} ions [31]. TF located on a phospholipid membrane enhances the catalytic activity of FVIIa for its natural substrates FIX and FX by approximately 10^7-fold [160]. TF also increases FVIIa activity in membrane-independent reactions with small substrates, although that increase is less pronounced than in membrane-dependent reactions. By using a fluorogenic substrate (6(Mes-D-Leu-Gly-Arg)amino-1-naphthalenediethylsulfamide), Lawson *et al.*, determined that the catalytic efficiency of substrate hydrolysis by FVIIa increases more than 100-fold when the FVIIa-TF complex is formed [161]. This increase in activity was suggested to be the result of a change in the FVIIa catalytic site allowing for a more efficient hydrolysis and an increase in the catalytic constant. The interaction or the hydrolysis rate was found to be independent of the supporting surface, with a Kd between 1.1–2.1 nM and enzyme:cofactor binding stoichiometry of 1:1. By using synthetic substrates, Butenas and coworkers determined that the amidolytic activity of the FVIIa–TF complex was greatly enhanced by the presence of Ca^{++} ions, with an observed Kd of the complex of 1.1 nM [31]. The presence of EDTA significantly decreased the amidolytic activity. It was observed that the formation of the complex does not require the presence of Ca^{++} ions, however in the absence of divalent cation, affinity and amidolytic activity of the complex is significantly reduced, suggesting that divalent metal ions are involved in cooperative interactions between FVIIa and TF.

Molecular Interactions of TF with FVIIa and FX

The zymogen FVII is converted efficiently to a functional serine protease only by the transmembrane domain-containing TF located on the membrane surface. A soluble form of TF, consisting of 219 residue long extracellular domain, can also serve as a cofactor in this reaction, although its efficiency is significantly reduced [162]. Factor VIIa consists of a light chain with γ-carboxyglutamic (Gla) and two epidermal growth factor (EGF)-like modules, which are covalently linked by a disulfide bridge to a serine protease domain in the heavy chain. Both chains bind to the extracellular region of TF (Fig. **4**) [163]. Mutagenesis studies allowed for further mapping of the molecular interaction of the TF-FVIIa complex. Fig. **4** highlights residues that are important for the molecular recognition of FVIIa and FX. An essential role for TF Lys165 and Lys166 in the activation of FX by the TF-FVIIa complex was assigned [164]. The allosteric disulfide bond between Cys186 and Cys209 is believed to facilitate a conformational change in the region where Lys165 and Lys166 are located allowing TF interaction with FX substrate (Fig. **4**). The FVIIa ligand binding site in TF extends over a broader region than in the proximity of the two lysines. Specific TF residues essential for the binding of FVIIa and the docking of FIX and FX have been mapped to be Lys20, Ile22, Glu24, Asp44, Trp45, Lys48, Asp58, Thr60, Phe76, Gln110, Arg135, Phe140 and Val207. These residues are primarily essential for binding of FVIIa ligand. Lysine 165, Lys166, Tyr157, Tyr158 and the disulfide bond between Cys186 and Cys209 are necessary for the structural component of TF and binding of FIX and FX. Binding of circulating FVIIa to TF establishes a base or docking site for FX by enhancing the interaction of TF and FX in close proximity to the phospholipid membrane [163].

Dimerization

The idea of TF dimerization originated out of an observation by Broze and coworkers that 20% of the protein became dimerized upon storage for several weeks in 2% Triton X-100 at -70C. Based on SDS-PAGE, the dimer exhibited an apparent molecular weight of 90 kDa [52]. Preliminary experiments suggested that the formation of the dimer has no effect on TF procoagulant activity. The notion that TF forms dimers on the surface of phopsholipid vesicles and cell membranes was also proposed by other investigators [165, 166]. Bach *et al.*, suggested that dimer formation occurs through the cytoplasmic half-cysteine and that the activity of the dimeric form is slightly lower than that of a monomeric form [165]. It was shown that purified human fibroblasts are modified by palmitate and stearate on the half-Cys245. Deacylation of that Cys245 during purification resulted in dimer formation. The existence of the heterodimer was observed by Carson without characterization of the band components[167]. Furthermore, Morrissey and coworkers observed heterodimerization of TF purified from human brain with the alpha chain of hemoglobin [168]. The heterodimer formation was suggested to be a secondary event to purification and occurred through a disulfide bond between the two proteins. A year later, Carson *et al.*, described the association to be coordinated through a disulfide involving the cytoplasmic domain Cys245 [169]. Therefore, it was concluded that dimer formation is an artifact of purification. It has been also shown that TF loses its tendency to dimerize in the absence of the cytoplasmic domain. Paborsky *et al.*, and Roy *et al.*, demonstrated that mutation of Cys245 reduced the tendency of TF to form dimers and that the transmembrane domain is essential for dimer formation [170, 171].

The phenomena of "encrypted" TF stems from observations that TF forms dimers. Bach *et al.*, suggested that TF exists in an encrypted dimeric form on the cell surface of HL-60 cells. This suggestion was based on the observation that dimerized TF demonstrated diminished procoagulant activity [172]. Upon stimulation with Ca^{++} ionophore, the dimers dissociated restoring procoagulant activity of TF. The authors suggested that dimer formation prevents the activation of FX by blocking FX interaction with the FVIIa-TF complex but has no effect on the binding of FVIIa to TF. Further support for this observation originated from a study by Le *et al.*, in which, according to the authors, the complex of FVIIa formed with TF expressed by the ovarian carcinoma cell line exhibited only 10-20% of expected procoagulant activity. The authors concluded that the remaining 80-90% of this complex existed in an encrypted dimerized form [173]. The proteolytic activity of the monomeric *versus* dimeric form of TF was later analyzed by Donate and coworkers with contradictory results [174]. Stable but reversible TF dimers were formed and expressed in BL21 *E. coli* cells. It was demonstrated that dimerization does not influence the amidolytic activity of the TF-FVIIa complex towards small substrates or the proteolytic activity towards FX. However it was suggested that TF dimerization greatly enhances the autoactivation of zymogen factor VII to FVIIa [174].

Posttranslational Modifications

Various forms of TF have been produced over the years and used to study the activity and function of TF. The expression systems exploited include insect cells, *E. coli*, yeast, and various mammalian cell lines. The quantities produced are larger than what could be isolated from natural sources and hence their popularity.

A major obstacle then arises as to the protein's genuine folding, activity and function granted different posttranslational modifications as per specific expression system. Limited work has been done on the contribution of each modification to the activity of TF and on the activity of the various sources of TF relative to each other. Recently more attention has been directed to the study of structure-function relationship of natural TF [57]. It seems a justifiable cause to investigate the influences of all these factors on TF function due to the threshold character (Fig. **5**) of the TF-triggered thrombin generation [175]. Seemingly minor changes in the specific TF activity may have profound effects on blood coagulation *in vivo*.

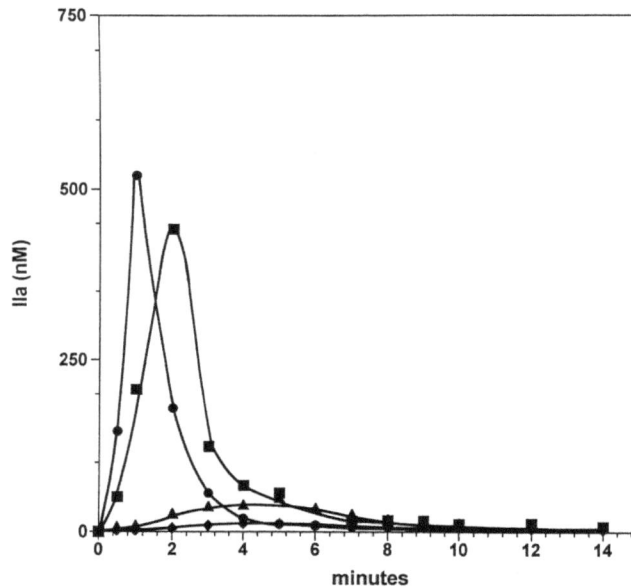

Figure 5: Thrombin generation by the TF-FVIIa complex. Varying concentrations of TF-FVIIa were used: 5 pM (♦), 10 pM (▲), 25 pM (■) and 125 pM (●). A dramatic change in thrombin generation is observed between 10 and 25 pM of TF-FVIIa. A small change in the TF-FVIIa concentration creates a threshold event with regards to thrombin generation. [This Figure was originally published in: van't Veer C, Mann KG. Regulation of tissue factor initiated thrombin generation by the stoichiometric inhibitors tissue factor pathway inhibitor, antithrombin-III, and heparin Cofactor-II. J Biol Chem 1992; 272(7): 4367-77 (see reference [175]).

Carbohydrates

Already in 1944, Chargaff *et al.*, was the first to observe the presence of carbohydrtaes in TF [143]. The sugar content constituted between 7-13% of total protein mass. Pitlick *et al.*, observed the binding of concanavalin A to thromboplastin protein and its inhibitory effect on the activity of the molecule [176]. A thorough study of the carbohydrate content of the thromboplastin protein was conducted by Bjorklid [50]. The analysis showed carbohydrate content of 6% composed of fucose, mannose, galactose and N-acetylneuranimidase. The somewhat acidic isoelectric point of the protein found to be between 5 and 6 was attributed to the presence of N-acetylneuranimidase. The linkage of the carbohydrate moiety to the TF backbone was presumed to be *via* asparagine. Paborsky determined the potential sites for TF glycosylation at Ans11, Asn124, Asn137 (Fig. **4**), all of which were within the recognized sequence for N-linked glycosylation, *i.e.* N-X-T/S [177]. The carbohydrates were reported to be insignificant for the coagulant activity of TF due to a similar activity of the non-glycosylated recombinant protein from *E. coli* and glycosylated one from kidney 293 cells. Rickles, Waxmann, Stone and their coworkers [178-180] also suggested that glycosylation is not required for full activity of TF. However, they suggested that glycosylation is required for the incorporation of TF into the cell membrane. In contrast, Pitlick, Shands, Bona and our data demonstrated that carbohydrates play a role in the activity of TF [57, 176, 181, 182]. Pitlick observed that concanavalin A inhibits the coagulant activity of TF by binding reversibly to the carbohydrate moiety of the protein. Shands and Bona both observed the loss of function and inability of TF to be incorporated into membranes after treatment with tunicamycin. Direct evidence for the effect of glycosylation on the activity of TF came from our laboratory when we compared the non-glycosylated rTF_{1-243} from *E.coli,* glycosylated rTF_{1-263} from Sf9 insect cells and natural TF from human placenta (pTF) in activity assays before and after treatment with glycosidases [57]. Our data showed that these forms of TF have different activities in both membrane independent fluorogenic assay and membrane dependent extrinsic FXase assay (Fig. **6**).

The amidolytic activity of the TF-FVIIa complex toward a fluorogenic substrate (membrane-independent assay) showed that the catalytic efficiency (Vmax) of the complex increased in the order $rTF_{1-243}<rTF_{1-263}<pTF$. Deglycosylation did not change the activity in this assay. In extrinsic FXase (membrane-dependent reaction), however, a 4-fold decrease in k_{cat} was observed for pTF-FVIIa upon deglycosylation, while the Km was minimally altered. After deglycosylation a small change in k_{cat} was observed for the rTF_{1-263}-FVIIa complex. The parameters of FX activation by both, deglycosylated rTF_{1-263}-FVIIa and pTF-FVIIa were similar to those of the non-glycosylated rTF_{1-243}-FVIIa. In conclusion, carbohydrates significantly influence the activity of natural TF in a physiologically relevant FX activation by the extrinsic FXase. Carbohydrate

analysis revealed glycosylation on Asn11, Asn124 and Asn137 in both rTF_{1-263} and pTF. The carbohydrates of rTF_{1-263} contain high-mannose, hybrid and fucosylated glycans. Natural pTF contains no high-mannose glycans but is modified with hybrid, highly fucosylated and sialylated sugars [57]. The extent of glycosylation on Asn11 is significantly different in the two proteins, *i.e.* 76% of pTF Asn11 is modified with glycans, whereas only 20% of Asn11 in rTF_{1-263} is glycosylated [183]. This suggests that not only composition but the extent of glycosylation may play a role in TF activity. Additionally, our study showed that 77% of rTF_{1-263} exists as a truncated protein missing the first two amino acids from the N-terminal end of the protein, whereas only 30% of pTF is in the truncated form. These observations indicate that structural components of recombinant TF proteins, specifically glycosylation, affect their activity and render them different form the natural counterpart.

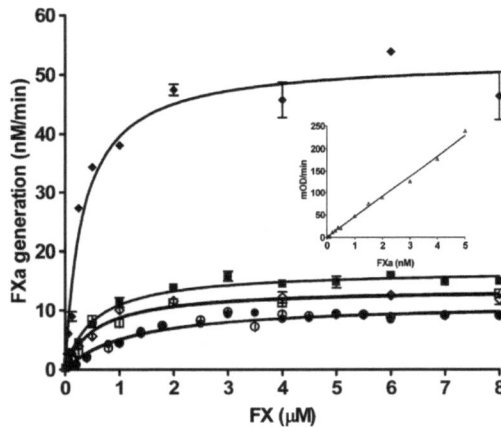

Figure 6: Extrinsic FXase assay. The graph shows the generation of FXa by glycosylated and deglycosylated TF in complex with FVIIa. The symbol (●) represents non-glycosylated rTF_{1-243} from *E.coli*, (○) represents rTF_{1-243} treated with glycosidase, (■) represents glysodylated rTF_{1-263} from Sf9 insect cells, (□) represents deglycosylated rTF_{1-263}, (♦) presents glycosylated from human placenta and (◊) represents deglycosylated pTF. FXa generation was measured and calculated from a FXa standard curve (inset). [This Figure was originally published in: Krudysz-Amblo *et al.*, Carbohydrates and activity of natural and recombinant tissue factor. J Biol Chem 2010; 285(5): 3371-3382. (see reference 57)].

Phosphorylation

Phosphorylation of the cytoplasmic domain of human TF has been reported [184]. Whether phosphorylation has an effect on TF function *in vivo* is not clear. *In vitro* studies showed that all three cytoplasmic serines (Ser)253, 258 and 263 in rTF may be phosphorylated [185]. Mody *et al.*, also reported *in vitro* phosphorylation of human placental TF on all three serines [185]. Serine 253 exhibits a consensus sequence Ser/Thr-X-Lys/Arg recognized by members of the protein kinase C (PKC), whereas Ser258 is not contained in the PKC recognition sequence, suggesting that it could be phosphorylated by a proline-directed kinase family [184]. The role of phosphorylation of the cytoplasmic domain of TF and its effect on TF procoagulant activity has been explored by various investigators and reviewed by Egorina and coworkers [186].

Cysteines and Disulfides

Tissue factor contains five cysteines; four of them (Cys49, Cys57, Cys186, Cys209) reside in the extracellular domain and one (Cys245) in the cytoplasmic domain. Two disulfide bridges between Cys49-Cys57 and Cys186-Cys209 have been reported (Fig. 4) [187]. Initially, Bach *et al.*, suggested that preservation of these disulfides is necessary for the full activity of TF [51]. Based on mutagenesis studies, a non-functional role has been assigned to N-terminal disulfide between Cys49-Cys57. Conversely, an important functional role has been assigned to the C-terminal disulfide between Cys186-Cys209 [187]. This assignment has been the subject of heated discussions in the scientific literature, although recent publications demonstrated that this disulfide bond is essential for TF function [188, 189]. The C-terminal cysteine bridge has been described as an allosteric disulfide [190]. An allosteric bond controls protein function by triggering conformational change upon its reduction or oxidation. Unlike the catalytic disulfide bond, which enzymatically mediates thiol-disulfide interchanges in substrate proteins, the allosteric bond, upon breaking or forming, nonenzymatically changes the intramolecular or intermolecular protein structure [191]. This bond in TF is solvent exposed, an atypical bond for the Fibronectin type III topology domains. The bond formed by Cys186 in the F strand to Cys209 in the adjacent G strand of the C module β-sheet is unusual, given the protein's secondary structure, *i.e.* a structure linked by noncovalent interactions between the antiparallel β-sheets. The two adjacent strands pucker to accommodate the disulfide bond. Due to such puckering, high potential energy may arise from the torsional energy and the deformation energy of the sheet [79]. Mutation of the C-terminal cysteines was shown to impair the procoagulant activity of TF [187, 192]. This has been suggested to account for the "encryption" theory in which TF exists in two forms on the cell surface: a minor population of active TF and a major population consisting of cryptic TF with significantly diminished activity [120]. The formation of the bond facilitates a conformational change of TF thus enhancing the binding of FVIIa and subsequent FX substrate activation. The mechanism of activation is believed to cause a reorientation of residues Tyr157,

Lys 159, Ser163, Gly 164, Lys165, Lys166 and Tyr185, which are important for binding of FX and FIX (Fig. **4**). Further enhancement of TF activity is caused by induced changes in Trp158-Lys159-Ser160 motif, which are important for substrate anchoring. Recently, protein disulfide isomerase (PDI) has been suggested as an important player in the formation and opening of the Cys186-Cys209 disulfide bond and consequently in the enhancement and reduction of activity, respectively. Ahamed *et al.*, postulates that PDI disrupts the bond and diminishes TF activity [193]. Reinhardt and coworkers report that PDI increases TF activity and fibrin generation [194]. Pendurthi and Kothari, both report lack of PDI influence on TF function [195, 196]. Popescu reviews the literature on PDI and TF activity and concludes that the topic itself remains "cryptic" [197]. In addition of two pairs of cysteines in the extracellular domain, there is one unpaired Cys in the COOH-terminus. It is linked to palmitate or stearate *via* a thioester bond [165], and it is not yet clear what direct role (if any) these modifications play in the procoagulant activity of TF.

OTHER ROLES OF TISSUE FACTOR

Tissue factor plays multiple roles in biological processes, with most of them being more or less closely related to coagulation. TF has been found to be important in cell signaling, cell migration and adhesion [198]. Intravascular processes initiated by TF have been linked to thrombosis, atherosclerosis, venous thromboembolism, cardiovascular and cerebrovascular diseases, hemophilia, diabetes, asthma, kidney disease, inflammation and cancer [44]. It has been postulated that the contribution of TF to arterial and venous thrombosis may be differential [199]. Arterial disease and cardiovascular risk factors have been attributed to some extent to circulating microparticles bearing TF [200]. Cardiovascular diseases, including stable coronary artery disease, stroke, acute coronary syndromes and pulmonary hypertension, have been correlated with increased concentration of circulating microparticles, specifically those of the platelet and endothelium origin [201]. Circulating leukocyte-derived microparticles have been suggested as a predictive marker of subclinical atherosclerosis burden [202]. The association between microparticles and arterial disease has been reviewed by Blann *et al.*, [203]. Inhibition of TF has been shown to reduce both arterial and venous thrombosis [204, 205]. Inhibition of the TF-FVIIa complex and FVIIa alone resulted in reduction of thrombus size [206, 207]. Vascular smooth muscle cells in the arterial wall have been shown to express TF [208]. Presence of TF has also been reported in atherosclerotic lesions [209]. Within the lesions, TF resides mainly in lipid areas, macrophages and smooth muscle cells determining plaque thrombogenicity [210]. After vascular injury, TF contributes to cell migration and remodeling [211]. In venous thrombosis, where thrombus formation is not associated with an injury of the vessel wall, the contribution of TF mainly comes from the protein presented on circulating microparticles [212].

An evidence for intracellular signaling through the cytoplasmic domain of TF has been suggested, although the TF-mediated signal transduction pathway has not been fully elucidated [213]. Recent studies describe a signaling cascade *via* a protease-activated receptor (PAR), where TF-bound FVIIa proteolytically activates the G-protein coupled receptors [44]. Ryden and coworkers reported that TF and PAR2 is upregulated in invasive tumors [214]. Schaffner *et al.*, showed that a crosstalk between the cytoplasmic domain of TF and PAR2 receptor occurs in angiogenic responses in breast cancer cells [215]. Vidwan and coworkers demonstrated that TF-induced thrombin generation on human aortic smooth muscle cells is regulated through activated PAR3 and PAR4 receptors, which play a significant role in the initiation phase of thrombin generation [216]. Demetz and coworkers described a link between the TF-FVIIa complex, PAR1 and PAR2 activation and inflammation [217]. The study showed that FVIIa induced IL-6 and IL-8 expression on smooth muscle cells, which correlated with increased expression of TF and PAR2. The proinflammatory effect was absent from endothelial and mononuclear cells. Additionally, the study suggested that elevated expression of PAR1, PAR2 and IL8 in atherosclerotic lesions confirms the interaction of TF and PARs in inflammation and atherosclerosis. So *et al.*, described a cross-talk between coagulation and inflammation [218]. Communication between these two systems has been described by other investigators as well [219, 220]. Inflammatory mediators such as cytokines (TNF-α and interleukins 1 and 6), chemokines, C-reactive protein and complement activation may stimulate TF-dependent coagulation in various ways. The common pathway is through the induction of TF expression on cells and its release in the form of microparticles. Disruption of the lipid bilayer in the endothelium and intravascular cells by inflammatory mediators leads to surface-exposed TF and contributes to the initiation of coagulation. Expression of specific markers of endothelium on released microparticles has been associated with endothelium-dependent coronary vasodilation [221]. A significant increase in monocytic TF mRNA has been noted in healthy subjects induced with endotoxemia [105]. Blocking TF activity inhibited inflammation-induced thrombin generation [219]. Inflammation may also promote coagulation through increased expression of leukocyte adhesion molecules on intravascular cell surfaces leading to activation of coagulation proteins. The interplay between inflammation, sepsis and coagulation has been also suggested [106, 222].

It has been recognized for a long time that coagulation activation occurs in cancer patients. Hematogenous tumor dissemination and growth of tumors has been attributed to an increased expression of TF [223]. Thrombin generation leads to enhanced interactions between tumor cells, vascular cells, platelets and endothelium through the augmentation of adhesion molecule expression [224]. Encapsulation of tumor cells in a fibrin and platelet rich clot may then initiate a plug of microcirculation [224]. Nash *et al.*, and Belting *et al.*, attributed TF activity in cancer specifically to its role in tumor angiogenesis and TF-mediated cellular signaling [225, 226]. Abe *et al.*, observed a correlation between overexpressed TF, increased vascular endothelial growth factor and decreased anti-angiogenic factor thrombospondin [227]. Clinically, the association of TF with microvessel density, a marker for tumor angiogenesis, supports this observation [228]. TF has been described as a marker of tumor progression and is believed to have a prometastatic function [229]. The association between TF expression and malignancy has been observed in many types of tumors [230-232]. In general, tumor-related TF expression coincides with thrombosis, metastasis, tumor progression and angiogenesis [233].

CONCLUSION

1. ACS patients have elevated levels of TF circulating in their blood.

2. TF is a non-enzymatic trans-membrane protein and is a key initiator of blood coagulation *in vivo*.

3. TF binds a serine protease (factor VIIa) and forms the extrinsic factor Xase complex on the membrane surface.

4. Formation of an extrinsic factor Xase increases proteolytic activity of factor VIIa by 7-9 orders of magnitude.

5. Post-translational modifications, particularly glycosylation, have a pronounced effect on the function of natural TF.

6. An allosteric disulfide bond Cys186-Cys209 is essential for TF function.

7. TF plays a role in cell signaling, migration and adhesion, and has been linked to thrombosis, atherosclerosis and venous thromboembolism.

8.   A correlation between TF expression and tumor malignancy, progression and angiogenesis has been observed.

ACKNOWLEDGMENTS

This work was supported by grant P01 HL46703 from the National Institutes of Health.

CONFLICT OF INTEREST

Kenneth Mann is consultant for Baxter. He has received honoraria from Bayer and is Chairman of the Board of Haematologic Technologies.

REFERENCES

[1]   Worthley SG, Osende JI, Helft G, Badimon JJ, Fuster V. Coronary artery disease: pathogenesis and acute coronary syndromes. Mt Sinai J Med. 2001; 68: 167-81.

[2]   Carter AM. Inflammation, thrombosis and acute coronary syndromes. Diab Vasc Dis Res. 2005; 2: 113-21.

[3]   Bevilacqua MP, Pober JS, Majeau GR, Fiers W, Cotran RS, Gimbrone MA, Jr. Recombinant tumor necrosis factor induces procoagulant activity in cultured human vascular endothelium: characterization and comparison with the actions of interleukin 1. Proc Natl Acad Sci U S A. 1986; 83: 4533-7.

[4]   Butenas S, Undas A, Gissel MT, Szuldrzynski K, Zmudka K, Mann KG. Factor XIa and tissue factor activity in patients with coronary artery disease. Thromb Haemost. 2008; 99: 142-9.

[5]   Kim HK, Song KS, Park YS, Yun YS, Shim WH. Changes of plasma tissue factor and tissue factor pathway inhibitor antigen levels and induction of tissue factor expression on the monocytes in coronary artery disease. Cardiology. 2000; 93: 31-6.

[6]   Saigo M, Abe S, Ogawa M, Yamashita T, Biro S, Minagoe S, Maruyama I, Tei C. Imbalance of plasminogen activator inhibitor-I/ tissue plasminogen activator and tissue factor/tissue factor pathway inhibitor in young Japanese men with myocardial infarction. Thromb Haemost. 2001; 86: 1197-203.

[7]   Andrie RP, Bauriedel G, Braun P, Hopp HW, Nickenig G, Skowasch D. Increased expression of C-reactive protein and tissue factor in acute coronary syndrome lesions: Correlation with serum C-reactive protein, angioscopic findings, and modification by statins. Atherosclerosis. 2009; 202: 135-43.

[8]   Bis J, Vojacek J, Dusek J, Pecka M, Palicka V, Stasek J, Maly J. Time-course of tissue factor plasma level in patients with acute coronary syndrome. Physiol Res. 2009; 58: 661-7.

[9]   Sakai T, Inoue S, Takei M, Ogawa G, Hamazaki Y, Ota H, Koboyashi Y. Activated inflammatory cells participate in thrombus size through tissue factor and plasminogen activator inhibitor-1 in acute coronary syndrome: Immunohistochemical analysis. Thromb Res. 2011; 127: 443-9.

[10]   Abdullah WZ, Moufak SK, Yusof Z, Mohamad MS, Kamarul IM. Shortened activated partial thromboplastin time, a hemostatic marker for hypercoagulable state during acute coronary event. Transl Res. 2010; 155: 315-9.

[11]   Brummel-Ziedins K, Undas A, Orfeo T, Gissel M, Butenas S, Zmudka K, Mann KG. Thrombin generation in acute coronary syndrome and stable coronary artery disease: dependence on plasma factor composition. J Thromb Haemost. 2008; 6: 104-10.

[12]   Folsom AR, Wu KK, Davis CE, Conlan MG, Sorlie PD, Szklo M. Population correlates of plasma fibrinogen and factor VII, putative cardiovascular risk factors. Atherosclerosis. 1991; 91: 191-205.

[13]   Green D, Chamberlain MA, Ruth KJ, Folsom AR, Liu K. Factor VII, cholesterol, and triglycerides. The CARDIA Study. Coronary Artery Risk Development in Young Adults Study. Arterioscler Thromb Vasc Biol. 1997; 17: 51-5.

[14]   Hong X, Shan PR, Hu L, Huang ZQ, Wu GJ, Xiao FY, Huang WJ. [Relationship between antithrombin-III value with acute coronary syndrome and preprocedural TIMI flow grade]. Zhonghua Yi Xue Za Zhi. 2012; 92: 831-4.

[15]   Pinelli A, Trivulzio S, Rossoni G, Redaelli R, Brenna S. Factors involved in sudden coagulation observed in patients with acute myocardial infarction. In Vivo. 2012; 26: 1021-5.

[16]   Bux-Gewehr I, Nacke A, Feurle GE. Recurring myocardial infarction in a 35 year old woman. Heart. 1999; 81: 316-7.

[17]   Sakata T, Kario K, Katayama Y, Matsuyama T, Kato H, Miyata T. Analysis of 45 episodes of arterial occlusive disease in Japanese patients with congenital protein C deficiency. Thromb Res. 1999; 94: 69-78.

[18]   Maly M, Vojacek J, Hrabos V, Kvasnicka J, Salaj P, Durdil V. Tissue factor, tissue factor pathway inhibitor and cytoadhesive molecules in patients with an acute coronary syndrome. Physiol Res. 2003; 52: 719-28.

[19]   Morange PE, Blankenberg S, Alessi MC, Bickel C, Rupprecht HJ, Schnabel R, Lubos E, Munzel T, Peetz D, Nicaud V, Juhan-Vague I, Tiret L. Prognostic value of plasma tissue factor and tissue factor pathway inhibitor for cardiovascular death in patients with coronary artery disease: the AtheroGene study. J Thromb Haemost. 2007; 5: 475-82.

[20]   Skeppholm M, Kallner A, Malmqvist K, Blomback M, Wallen H. Is fibrin formation and thrombin generation increased during and after an acute coronary syndrome? Thromb Res. 2011; 128: 483-9.

[21]   Lu D, Owens J, Kreutz RP. Plasma and Whole Blood Clot Strength Measured by Thrombelastography in Patients Treated with Clopidogrel during Acute Coronary Syndromes. Thromb Res. 2013; 132: e94-8.

[22]   Abbate R, Cioni G, Ricci I, Miranda M, Gori AM. Thrombosis and acute coronary syndrome. Thromb Res. 2012; 129: 235-40.

[23]   Meade TW, Ruddock V, Stirling Y, Chakrabarti R, Miller GJ. Fibrinolytic activity, clotting factors, and long-term incidence of ischaemic heart disease in the Northwick Park Heart Study. Lancet. 1993; 342: 1076-9.

[24]   Hamsten A, de Faire U, Walldius G, Dahlen G, Szamosi A, Landou C, Blomback M, Wiman B. Plasminogen activator inhibitor in plasma: risk factor for recurrent myocardial infarction. Lancet. 1987; 2: 3-9.

[25]   Spicer EK, Horton R, Bloem L, Bach R, Williams KR, Guha A, Kraus J, Lin TC, Nemerson Y, Konigsberg WH. Isolation of cDNA clones coding for human tissue factor: primary structure of the protein and cDNA. Proc Natl Acad Sci U S A. 1987; 84: 5148-52.

[26]   Toomey JR, Kratzer KE, Lasky NM, Stanton JJ, Broze GJ, Jr. Targeted disruption of the murine tissue factor gene results in embryonic lethality. Blood. 1996; 88: 1583-7.

[27]   Krishnaswamy S, Field KA, Edgington TS, Morrissey JH, Mann KG. Role of the membrane surface in the activation of human coagulation factor X. J Biol Chem. 1992; 267: 26110-20.

[28]   Mann KG. Thrombin formation. Chest. 2003; 124: 4S-10S.

[29]   Mann KG, Orfeo T, Butenas S, Undas A, Brummel-Ziedins K. Blood coagulation dynamics in haemostasis. Hamostaseologie. 2009; 29: 7-16.

[30]   Butenas S, Mann KG. Kinetics of human factor VII activation. Biochemistry. 1996; 35: 1904-10.

[31]   Butenas S, Lawson JH, Kalafatis M, Mann KG. Cooperative interaction of divalent metal ions, substrate, and tissue factor with factor VIIa. Biochemistry. 1994; 33: 3449-56.

[32]   Butenas S, Orfeo T, Brummel-Ziedins KE, Mann KG. Tissue factor in thrombosis and hemorrhage. Surgery. 2007; 142: S2-14.

[33]   Butenas S, Orfeo T, Mann KG. Tissue factor activity and function in blood coagulation. Thromb Res. 2008; 122 Suppl 1: S42-6.

[34]   Mackman N, Tilley RE, Key NS. Role of the extrinsic pathway of blood coagulation in hemostasis and thrombosis. Arterioscler Thromb Vasc Biol. 2007; 27: 1687-93.

[35]   Gailani D, Renne T. Intrinsic pathway of coagulation and arterial thrombosis. Arterioscler Thromb Vasc Biol. 2007; 27: 2507-13.

[36]   Jowett B. The dialogues of Plato. New York: Macmillan, 1892.

[37]   Lee HDP. Aristotle: Meterologica. Cambridge: Harvard University Press, 1952.

[38]   Martin DM, Wiiger MT, Prydz H. Tissue factor and biotechnology. Thromb Res. 1998; 90: 1-25.

[39]   Mills CA. Chemical nature of tissue coagulins. J Biol Chem. 1921; 46: 135-65.

[40]　Wooldridge LC. On the chemistry of blood and other scientific papers. London: Kegan Paul, 1893.

[41]　Camerer E, Kolsto AB, Prydz H. Cell biology of tissue factor, the principal initiator of blood coagulation. Thromb Res. 1996; 81: 1-41.

[42]　Howell WH. The nature and action of the thromboplastic (zymoplastic) substance of the tissues. Am J Physiol. 1912; 31: 1-21.

[43]　Chargaff E. Studies on the mechanism of the thromboplastic effect. J Biol Chem. 1948; 173: 253-62.

[44]　Mackman N. The many faces of tissue factor. J Thromb Haemost. 2009; 7 Suppl 1: 136-9.

[45]　Cohen SS, Chargaff E. Studies on the chemistry of blood coagulation: IX. The thromboplastic protein from lungs. J Biol Chem. 1940; 136: 243-56.

[46]　Chargaff E, Moore DH, Bendich A. Ultracentrifugal isolation from lung tissue of a macromolecular protein component with thromboplastic properties. J Biol Chem. 1942; 145: 593-603.

[47]　Bjorklid E, Storm E, Osterud B, Prydz H. The interaction of the protein and phospholipid components of tissue thromboplastin (factor III) with the factors VII and X. Scand J Haematol. 1975; 14: 65-70.

[48]　Pitlick FA, Nemerson Y. Purification and characterization of tissue factor apoprotein. Methods Enzymol. 1976; 45: 37-48.

[49]　Liu DT, McCoy LE. Tissue extract thromboplastin: quantitation, fractionation and characterization of protein components. Thromb Res. 1975; 7: 199.

[50]　Bjorklid E, Storm E. Purification and some properties of the protein component of tissue thromboplastin from human brain. Biochem J. 1977; 165: 89-96.

[51]　Bach R, Nemerson Y, Konigsberg W. Purification and characterization of bovine tissue factor. J Biol Chem. 1981; 256: 8324-31.

[52]　Broze GJ, Jr., Leykam JE, Schwartz BD, Miletich JP. Purification of human brain tissue factor. J Biol Chem. 1985; 260: 10917-20.

[53]　Guha A, Bach R, Konigsberg W, Nemerson Y. Affinity purification of human tissue factor: interaction of factor VII and tissue factor in detergent micelles. Proc Natl Acad Sci U S A. 1986; 83: 299-302.

[54]　Cohen SS, Chargaff E. Studies on the chemistry of blood coagulation: XIII. The phosphatide constituents of the thromboplastic protein from lungs. J Biol Chem. 1941; 139: 741-52.

[55]　Cohen SS, Chargaff E. The electrophoretic properties of the thromboplastic protein from lungs. J Biol Chem. 1941; 140: 689-95.

[56]　Bjorklid E, Storm E, Prydz H. The protein component of human brain thromboplastin. Biochem Biophys Res Commun. 1973; 55: 969-76.

[57]　Krudysz-Amblo J, Jennings ME, 2nd, Mann KG, Butenas S. Carbohydrates and activity of natural and recombinant tissue factor. J Biol Chem. 2010; 285: 3371-82.

[58]　Scarpati EM, Wen D, Broze GJ, Jr., Miletich JP, Flandermeyer RR, Siegel NR, Sadler JE. Human tissue factor: cDNA sequence and chromosome localization of the gene. Biochemistry. 1987; 26: 5234-8.

[59]　Kao FT, Hartz J, Horton R, Nemerson Y, Carson SD. Regional assignment of human tissue factor gene (F3) to chromosome 1p21-p22. Somat Cell Mol Genet. 1988; 14: 407-10.

[60]　Morrissey JH, Fakhrai H, Edgington TS. Molecular cloning of the cDNA for tissue factor, the cellular receptor for the initiation of the coagulation protease cascade. Cell. 1987; 50: 129-35.

[61]　Fisher KL, Gorman CM, Vehar GA, O'Brien DP, Lawn RM. Cloning and expression of human tissue factor cDNA. Thromb Res. 1987; 48: 89-99.

[62]　Mackman N, Morrissey JH, Fowler B, Edgington TS. Complete sequence of the human tissue factor gene, a highly regulated cellular receptor that initiates the coagulation protease cascade. Biochemistry. 1989; 28: 1755-62.

[63]　Takayenoki Y, Muta T, Miyata T, Iwanaga S. cDNA and amino acid sequences of bovine tissue factor. Biochem Biophys Res Commun. 1991; 181: 1145-50.

[64]　Ranganathan G, Blatti SP, Subramaniam M, Fass DN, Maihle NJ, Getz MJ. Cloning of murine tissue factor and regulation of gene expression by transforming growth factor type beta 1. J Biol Chem. 1991; 266: 496-501.

[65]　Taby O, Rosenfield CL, Bogdanov V, Nemerson Y, Taubman MB. Cloning of the rat tissue factor cDNA and promoter: identification of a serum-response region. Thromb Haemost. 1996; 76: 697-702.

[66]　Pawashe A, Ezekowitz M, Lin TC, Horton R, Bach R, Konigsberg W. Molecular cloning, characterization and expression of cDNA for rabbit brain tissue factor. Thromb Haemost. 1991; 66: 315-20.

[67]   Kadonaga JT, Jones KA, Tjian R. Promoter-specific activation of RNA polymerase II transcription by Sp1. Trends Biochem Sci. 1986; 11: 20-3.

[68]   Berg JM. Sp1 and the subfamily of zinc finger proteins with guanine-rich binding sites. Proc Natl Acad Sci U S A. 1992; 89: 11109-10.

[69]   Lee W, Mitchell P, Tjian R. Purified transcription factor AP-1 interacts with TPA-inducible enhancer elements. Cell. 1987; 49: 741-52.

[70]   Imagawa M, Chiu R, Karin M. Transcription factor AP-2 mediates induction by two different signal-transduction pathways: protein kinase C and cAMP. Cell. 1987; 51: 251-60.

[71]   Singh H, LeBowitz JH, Baldwin AS, Jr., Sharp PA. Molecular cloning of an enhancer binding protein: isolation by screening of an expression library with a recognition site DNA. Cell. 1988; 52: 415-23.

[72]   Mackman N, Fowler BJ, Edgington TS, Morrissey JH. Functional analysis of the human tissue factor promoter and induction by serum. Proc Natl Acad Sci U S A. 1990; 87: 2254-8.

[73]   Bazan JF. Structural design and molecular evolution of a cytokine receptor superfamily. Proc Natl Acad Sci U S A. 1990; 87: 6934-8.

[74]   de Vos AM, Ultsch M, Kossiakoff AA. Human growth hormone and extracellular domain of its receptor: crystal structure of the complex. Science. 1992; 255: 306-12.

[75]   Somers W, Ultsch M, De Vos AM, Kossiakoff AA. The X-ray structure of a growth hormone-prolactin receptor complex. Nature. 1994; 372: 478-81.

[76]   Livnah O, Stura EA, Johnson DL, Middleton SA, Mulcahy LS, Wrighton NC, Dower WJ, Jolliffe LK, Wilson IA. Functional mimicry of a protein hormone by a peptide agonist: the EPO receptor complex at 2.8 A. Science. 1996; 273: 464-71.

[77]   Walter MR, Windsor WT, Nagabhushan TL, Lundell DJ, Lunn CA, Zauodny PJ, Narula SK. Crystal structure of a complex between interferon-gamma and its soluble high-affinity receptor. Nature. 1995; 376: 230-5.

[78]   Bodian DL, Jones EY, Harlos K, Stuart DI, Davis SJ. Crystal structure of the extracellular region of the human cell adhesion molecule CD2 at 2.5 A resolution. Structure. 1994; 2: 755-66.

[79]   Harlos K, Martin DM, O'Brien DP, Jones EY, Stuart DI, Polikarpov I, Miller A, Tuddenham EG, Boys CW. Crystal structure of the extracellular region of human tissue factor. Nature. 1994; 370: 662-6.

[80]   Quirk SM, Pentecost BT, Mackman N, Loskutoff DJ, Hartzell S, Henrikson KP. The regulation of uterine tissue factor by estrogen. Endocrine. 1995; 3: 177-84.

[81]   Luther T, Flossel C, Mackman N, Bierhaus A, Kasper M, Albrecht S, Sage EH, Iruela-Arispe L, Grossmann H, Strohlein A, Zhang Y, Nawroth PP, Carmeliet P, Loskutoff DJ, Muller M. Tissue factor expression during human and mouse development. Am J Pathol. 1996; 149: 101-13.

[82]   Baron M, Main AL, Driscoll PC, Mardon HJ, Boyd J, Campbell ID. 1H NMR assignment and secondary structure of the cell adhesion type III module of fibronectin. Biochemistry. 1992; 31: 2068-73.

[83]   Dean DC, Bowlus CL, Bourgeois S. Cloning and analysis of the promotor region of the human fibronectin gene. Proc Natl Acad Sci U S A. 1987; 84: 1876-80.

[84]   Peppelenbosch MP, Versteeg HH. Cell biology of tissue factor, an unusual member of the cytokine receptor family. Trends Cardiovasc Med. 2001; 11: 335-9.

[85]   Astrup T. Assay and content of tissue thromboplastin in different organs. Thromb Diath Haemorrh. 1965; 14: 401-16.

[86]   Drake TA, Morrissey JH, Edgington TS. Selective cellular expression of tissue factor in human tissues. Implications for disorders of hemostasis and thrombosis. Am J Pathol. 1989; 134: 1087-97.

[87]   Faulk WP, Labarrere CA, Carson SD. Tissue factor: identification and characterization of cell types in human placentae. Blood. 1990; 76: 86-96.

[88]   Fleck RA, Rao LV, Rapaport SI, Varki N. Localization of human tissue factor antigen by immunostaining with monospecific, polyclonal anti-human tissue factor antibody. Thromb Res. 1990; 59: 421-37.

[89]   Lockwood CJ, Nemerson Y, Guller S, Krikun G, Alvarez M, Hausknecht V, Gurpide E, Schatz F. Progestational regulation of human endometrial stromal cell tissue factor expression during decidualization. J Clin Endocrinol Metab. 1993; 76: 231-6.

[90]   Bouchard BA, Shatos MA, Tracy PB. Human brain pericytes differentially regulate expression of procoagulant enzyme complexes comprising the extrinsic pathway of blood coagulation. Arterioscler Thromb Vasc Biol. 1997; 17: 1-9.

[91]   Schecter AD, Spirn B, Rossikhina M, Giesen PL, Bogdanov V, Fallon JT, Fisher EA, Schnapp LM, Nemerson Y, Taubman MB. Release of active tissue factor by human arterial smooth muscle cells. Circ Res. 2000; 87: 126-32.

[92]   Flossel C, Luther T, Muller M, Albrecht S, Kasper M. Immunohistochemical detection of tissue factor (TF) on paraffin sections of routinely fixed human tissue. Histochemistry. 1994; 101: 449-53.

[93]   Solovey A, Gui L, Key NS, Hebbel RP. Tissue factor expression by endothelial cells in sickle cell anemia. J Clin Invest. 1998; 101: 1899-904.

[94]   Contrino J, Hair G, Kreutzer DL, Rickles FR. In situ detection of tissue factor in vascular endothelial cells: correlation with the malignant phenotype of human breast disease. Nat Med. 1996; 2: 209-15.

[95]   Hair GA, Padula S, Zeff R, Schmeizl M, Contrino J, Kreutzer DL, de Moerloose P, Boyd AW, Stanley I, Burgess AW, Rickles FR. Tissue factor expression in human leukemic cells. Leuk Res. 1996; 20: 1-11.

[96]   Thiruvikraman SV, Guha A, Roboz J, Taubman MB, Nemerson Y, Fallon JT. In situ localization of tissue factor in human atherosclerotic plaques by binding of digoxigenin-labeled factors VIIa and X. Lab Invest. 1996; 75: 451-61.

[97]   More L, Sim R, Hudson M, Dhillon AP, Pounder R, Wakefield AJ. Immunohistochemical study of tissue factor expression in normal intestine and idiopathic inflammatory bowel disease. J Clin Pathol. 1993; 46: 703-8.

[98]   Parry GC, Mackman N. Transcriptional regulation of tissue factor expression in human endothelial cells. Arterioscler Thromb Vasc Biol. 1995; 15: 612-21.

[99]   Szotowski B, Antoniak S, Poller W, Schultheiss HP, Rauch U. Procoagulant soluble tissue factor is released from endothelial cells in response to inflammatory cytokines. Circ Res. 2005; 96: 1233-9.

[100]   Marchetti M, Vignoli A, Bani MR, Balducci D, Barbui T, Falanga A. All-trans retinoic acid modulates microvascular endothelial cell hemostatic properties. Haematologica. 2003; 88: 895-905.

[101]   Sturk-Maquelin KN, Nieuwland R, Romijn FP, Eijsman L, Hack CE, Sturk A. Pro- and non-coagulant forms of non-cell-bound tissue factor in vivo. J Thromb Haemost. 2003; 1: 1920-6.

[102]   Osterud B. Tissue factor expression in blood cells. Thromb Res. 2010; 125 Suppl 1: S31-4.

[103]   Campbell JE, Brummel-Ziedins KE, Butenas S, Mann KG. Cellular regulation of blood coagulation: a model for venous stasis. Blood. 2010; 116: 6082-91.

[104]   Gregory SA, Morrissey JH, Edgington TS. Regulation of tissue factor gene expression in the monocyte procoagulant response to endotoxin. Mol Cell Biol. 1989; 9: 2752-5.

[105]   Franco RF, de Jonge E, Dekkers PE, Timmerman JJ, Spek CA, van Deventer SJ, van Deursen P, van Kerkhoff L, van Gemen B, ten Cate H, van der Poll T, Reitsma PH. The in vivo kinetics of tissue factor messenger RNA expression during human endotoxemia: relationship with activation of coagulation. Blood. 2000; 96: 554-9.

[106]   Esmon CT, Fukudome K, Mather T, Bode W, Regan LM, Stearns-Kurosawa DJ, Kurosawa S. Inflammation, sepsis, and coagulation. Haematologica. 1999; 84: 254-9.

[107]   Ritis K, Doumas M, Mastellos D, Micheli A, Giaglis S, Magotti P, Rafail S, Kartalis G, Sideras P, Lambris JD. A novel C5a receptor-tissue factor cross-talk in neutrophils links innate immunity to coagulation pathways. J Immunol. 2006; 177: 4794-802.

[108]   Scharf RE, Tomer A, Marzec UM, Teirstein PS, Ruggeri ZM, Harker LA. Activation of platelets in blood perfusing angioplasty-damaged coronary arteries. Flow cytometric detection. Arterioscler Thromb. 1992; 12: 1475-87.

[109]   Satta N, Toti F, Feugeas O, Bohbot A, Dachary-Prigent J, Eschwege V, Hedman H, Freyssinet JM. Monocyte vesiculation is a possible mechanism for dissemination of membrane-associated procoagulant activities and adhesion molecules after stimulation by lipopolysaccharide. J Immunol. 1994; 153: 3245-55.

[110]   Mallat Z, Hugel B, Ohan J, Leseche G, Freyssinet JM, Tedgui A. Shed membrane microparticles with procoagulant potential in human atherosclerotic plaques: a role for apoptosis in plaque thrombogenicity. Circulation. 1999; 99: 348-53.

[111]   Combes V, Simon AC, Grau GE, Arnoux D, Camoin L, Sabatier F, Mutin M, Sanmarco M, Sampol J, Dignat-George F. In vitro generation of endothelial microparticles and possible prothrombotic activity in patients with lupus anticoagulant. J Clin Invest. 1999; 104: 93-102.

[112]   Piccin A, Murphy WG, Smith OP. Circulating microparticles: pathophysiology and clinical implications. Blood Rev. 2007; 21: 157-71.

[113]   Aras O, Shet A, Bach RR, Hysjulien JL, Slungaard A, Hebbel RP, Escolar G, Jilma B, Key NS. Induction of microparticle- and cell-associated intravascular tissue factor in human endotoxemia. Blood. 2004; 103: 4545-53.

[114]   Shet AS, Aras O, Gupta K, Hass MJ, Rausch DJ, Saba N, Koopmeiners L, Key NS, Hebbel RP. Sickle blood contains tissue factor-positive microparticles derived from endothelial cells and monocytes. Blood. 2003; 102: 2678-83.

[115]   Tesselaar ME, Romijn FP, Van Der Linden IK, Prins FA, Bertina RM, Osanto S. Microparticle-associated tissue factor activity: a link between cancer and thrombosis? J Thromb Haemost. 2007; 5: 520-7.

[116]   Rauch U, Antoniak S. Tissue factor-positive microparticles in blood associated with coagulopathy in cancer. Thromb Haemost. 2007; 97: 9-10.

[117]   Furie B, Furie BC. Role of platelet P-selectin and microparticle PSGL-1 in thrombus formation. Trends Mol Med. 2004; 10: 171-8.

[118]   Aharon A, Tamari T, Brenner B. Monocyte-derived microparticles and exosomes induce procoagulant and apoptotic effects on endothelial cells. Thromb Haemost. 2008; 100: 878-85.

[119]   Sabatier F, Roux V, Anfosso F, Camoin L, Sampol J, Dignat-George F. Interaction of endothelial microparticles with monocytic cells in vitro induces tissue factor-dependent procoagulant activity. Blood. 2002; 99: 3962-70.

[120]   Bach RR. Tissue factor encryption. Arterioscler Thromb Vasc Biol. 2006; 26: 456-61.

[121]   Essayagh S, Xuereb JM, Terrisse AD, Tellier-Cirioni L, Pipy B, Sie P. Microparticles from apoptotic monocytes induce transient platelet recruitment and tissue factor expression by cultured human vascular endothelial cells via a redox-sensitive mechanism. Thromb Haemost. 2007; 98: 831-7.

[122]   Rauch U, Bonderman D, Bohrmann B, Badimon JJ, Himber J, Riederer MA, Nemerson Y. Transfer of tissue factor from leukocytes to platelets is mediated by CD15 and tissue factor. Blood. 2000; 96: 170-5.

[123]   Banfi C, Brioschi M, Wait R, Begum S, Gianazza E, Pirillo A, Mussoni L, Tremoli E. Proteome of endothelial cell-derived procoagulant microparticles. Proteomics. 2005; 5: 4443-55.

[124]   Diamant M, Tushuizen ME, Abid-Hussein MN, Hau CM, Boing AN, Sturk A, Nieuwland R. Simvastatin-induced endothelial cell detachment and microparticle release are prenylation dependent. Thromb Haemost. 2008; 100: 489-97.

[125]   Zillmann A, Luther T, Muller I, Kotzsch M, Spannagl M, Kauke T, Oelschlagel U, Zahler S, Engelmann B. Platelet-associated tissue factor contributes to the collagen-triggered activation of blood coagulation. Biochem Biophys Res Commun. 2001; 281: 603-9.

[126]   Muller I, Klocke A, Alex M, Kotzsch M, Luther T, Morgenstern E, Zieseniss S, Zahler S, Preissner K, Engelmann B. Intravascular tissue factor initiates coagulation via circulating microvesicles and platelets. FASEB J. 2003; 17: 476-8.

[127]   Panes O, Matus V, Saez CG, Quiroga T, Pereira J, Mezzano D. Human platelets synthesize and express functional tissue factor. Blood. 2007; 109: 5242-50.

[128]   Schwertz H, Tolley ND, Foulks JM, Denis MM, Risenmay BW, Buerke M, Tilley RE, Rondina MT, Harris EM, Kraiss LW, Mackman N, Zimmerman GA, Weyrich AS. Signal-dependent splicing of tissue factor pre-mRNA modulates the thrombogenicity of human platelets. J Exp Med. 2006; 203: 2433-40.

[129]   Camera M, Frigerio M, Toschi V, Brambilla M, Rossi F, Cottell DC, Maderna P, Parolari A, Bonzi R, De Vincenti O, Tremoli E. Platelet activation induces cell-surface immunoreactive tissue factor expression, which is modulated differently by antiplatelet drugs. Arterioscler Thromb Vasc Biol. 2003; 23: 1690-6.

[130]   Butenas S, Bouchard BA, Brummel-Ziedins KE, Parhami-Seren B, Mann KG. Tissue factor activity in whole blood. Blood. 2005; 105: 2764-70.

[131]   Osterud B, Bjorklid E. Sources of tissue factor. Semin Thromb Hemost. 2006; 32: 11-23.

[132]   Bouchard BA, Mann KG, Butenas S. No evidence for tissue factor on platelets. Blood. 2010; 116: 854-5.

[133]   Bogdanov VY, Balasubramanian V, Hathcock J, Vele O, Lieb M, Nemerson Y. Alternatively spliced human tissue factor: a circulating, soluble, thrombogenic protein. Nat Med. 2003; 9: 458-62.

[134]　Censarek P, Bobbe A, Grandoch M, Schror K, Weber AA. Alternatively spliced human tissue factor (asHTF) is not pro-coagulant. Thromb Haemost. 2007; 97: 11-4.

[135]　Hobbs JE, Zakarija A, Cundiff DL, Doll JA, Hymen E, Cornwell M, Crawford SE, Liu N, Signaevsky M, Soff GA. Alternatively spliced human tissue factor promotes tumor growth and angiogenesis in a pancreatic cancer tumor model. Thromb Res. 2007; 120 Suppl 2: S13-21.

[136]　Boing AN, Hau CM, Sturk A, Nieuwland R. Human alternatively spliced tissue factor is not secreted and does not trigger coagulation. J Thromb Haemost. 2009; 7: 1423-6.

[137]　Rand MD, Lock JB, van't Veer C, Gaffney DP, Mann KG. Blood clotting in minimally altered whole blood. Blood. 1996; 88: 3432-45.

[138]　Santucci RA, Erlich J, Labriola J, Wilson M, Kao KJ, Kickler TS, Spillert C, Mackman N. Measurement of tissue factor activity in whole blood. Thromb Haemost. 2000; 83: 445-54.

[139]　Parhami-Seren B, Butenas S, Krudysz-Amblo J, Mann KG. Immunologic quantitation of tissue factors. J Thromb Haemost. 2006; 4: 1747-55.

[140]　Bogdanov VY, Cimmino G, Tardos JG, Tunstead JR, Badimon JJ. Assessment of plasma tissue factor activity in patients presenting with coronary artery disease: limitations of a commercial assay. J Thromb Haemost. 2009; 7: 894-7.

[141]　Hvatum M, Prydz H. Studies on tissue thromboplastin--its splitting into two separable parts. Thromb Diath Haemorrh. 1969; 21: 217-22.

[142]　Nemerson Y. Characteristics and lipid requirements of coagulant proteins extracted from lung and brain: the specifity of protein component of tissue factor. J Clin Invest. 1969; 48: 322-31.

[143]　Chargaff E, Bendich A, Cohen SS. The thromboplastic protein: structure, properties, disintegration. J Biol Chem. 1944; 156: 161-78.

[144]　Pitlick FA, Nemerson Y. Binding of the protein component of tissue factor to phospholipids. Biochemistry. 1970; 9: 5105-13.

[145]　Liu DT, McCoy LE. Phospholipid requirements of tissue thromboplastin in blood coagulation. Thromb Res. 1975; 7: 213-21.

[146]　Nemerson Y. The phospholipid requirement of tissue factor in blood coagulation. J Clin Invest. 1968; 47: 72-80.

[147]　Bull RK, Jevons S, Barton PG. Complexes of prothrombin with calcium ions and phospholipids. J Biol Chem. 1972; 247: 2747-54.

[148]　Marcus AJ, Zucker-Franklin D, Safier LB, Ullman HL. Studies on human platelet granules and membranes. J Clin Invest. 1966; 45: 14-28.

[149]　Butenas S, Gissel M, Krudysz-Amblo J, Mann KG. The nature of lipopolysaccharide-stimulated monocyte tissue factor activity. Blood Coagul Fibrinolysis. 2013.

[150]　Esnouf MP, Williams WJ. The isolation and purification of a bovine-plasma protein which is a substrate for the coagulant fraction of Russell's-viper venom. Biochem J. 1962; 84: 62-71.

[151]　Nemerson Y, Spaet TH. The Activation of Factor X by Extracts of Rabbit Brain. Blood. 1964; 23: 657-68.

[152]　Williams WJ, Norris DG. Purification of a bovine plasma protein (factor VII) which is required for the activity of lung microsomes in blood coagulation. J Biol Chem. 1966; 241: 1847-56.

[153]　Nemerson Y. The reaction between bovine brain tissue factor and factors VII and X. Biochemistry. 1966; 5: 601-8.

[154]　Silverberg SA, Nemerson Y, Zur M. Kinetics of the activation of bovine coagulation factor X by components of the extrinsic pathway. Kinetic behavior of two-chain factor VII in the presence and absence of tissue factor. J Biol Chem. 1977; 252: 8481-8.

[155]　Osterud B, Rapaport SI. Activation of factor IX by the reaction product of tissue factor and factor VII: additional pathway for initiating blood coagulation. Proc Natl Acad Sci U S A. 1977; 74: 5260-4.

[156]　Nemerson Y, Esnouf MP. Activation of a proteolytic system by a membrane lipoprotein: mechanism of action of tissue factor. Proc Natl Acad Sci U S A. 1973; 70: 310-4.

[157]　Jesty J, Nemerson Y. Purification of Factor VII from bovine plasma. Reaction with tissue factor and activation of Factor X. J Biol Chem. 1974; 249: 509-15.

[158]　Lawson JH, Butenas S, Mann KG. The evaluation of complex-dependent alterations in human factor VIIa. J Biol Chem. 1992; 267: 4834-43.

[159]　Rao LV, Williams T, Rapaport SI. Studies of the activation of factor VII bound to tissue factor. Blood. 1996; 87: 3738-48.

[160]   Komiyama Y, Pedersen AH, Kisiel W. Proteolytic activation of human factors IX and X by recombinant human factor VIIa: effects of calcium, phospholipids, and tissue factor. Biochemistry. 1990; 29: 9418-25.

[161]   Lawson JH, Mann KG. Cooperative activation of human factor IX by the human extrinsic pathway of blood coagulation. J Biol Chem. 1991; 266: 11317-27.

[162]   Payne MA, Neuenschwander PF, Johnson AE, Morrissey JH. Effect of soluble tissue factor on the kinetic mechanism of factor VIIa: enhancement of p-guanidinobenzoate substrate hydrolysis. Biochemistry. 1996; 35: 7100-6.

[163]   Martin DM, Boys CW, Ruf W. Tissue factor: molecular recognition and cofactor function. FASEB J. 1995; 9: 852-9.

[164]   Huang Q, Neuenschwander PF, Rezaie AR, Morrissey JH. Substrate recognition by tissue factor-factor VIIa. Evidence for interaction of residues Lys165 and Lys166 of tissue factor with the 4-carboxyglutamate-rich domain of factor X. J Biol Chem. 1996; 271: 21752-7.

[165]   Bach R, Konigsberg WH, Nemerson Y. Human tissue factor contains thioester-linked palmitate and stearate on the cytoplasmic half-cystine. Biochemistry. 1988; 27: 4227-31.

[166]   Fair DS, MacDonald MJ. Cooperative interaction between factor VII and cell surface-expressed tissue factor. J Biol Chem. 1987; 262: 11692-8.

[167]   Carson SD. Continuous chromogenic tissue factor assay: comparison to clot-based assays and sensitivity established using pure tissue factor. Thromb Res. 1987; 47: 379-87.

[168]   Morrissey JH, Revak D, Tejada P, Fair DS, Edgington TS. Resolution of monomeric and heterodimeric forms of tissue factor, the high-affinity cellular receptor for factor VII. Thromb Res. 1988; 50: 481-93.

[169]   Carson SD, Ross SE, Gramzinski RA. Protein co-isolated with human tissue factor impairs recovery of activity. Blood. 1988; 71: 520-3.

[170]   Paborsky LR, Tate KM, Harris RJ, Yansura DG, Band L, McCray G, Gorman CM, O'Brien DP, Chang JY, Swartz JR, et al. Purification of recombinant human tissue factor. Biochemistry. 1989; 28: 8072-7.

[171]   Roy S, Paborsky LR, Vehar GA. Self-association of tissue factor as revealed by chemical crosslinking. J Biol Chem. 1991; 266: 4665-8.

[172]   Bach RR, Moldow CF. Mechanism of tissue factor activation on HL-60 cells. Blood. 1997; 89: 3270-6.

[173]   Le DT, Rapaport SI, Rao LV. Relations between factor VIIa binding and expression of factor VIIa/tissue factor catalytic activity on cell surfaces. J Biol Chem. 1992; 267: 15447-54.

[174]   Donate F, Kelly CR, Ruf W, Edgington TS. Dimerization of tissue factor supports solution-phase autoactivation of factor VII without influencing proteolytic activation of factor X. Biochemistry. 2000; 39: 11467-76.

[175]   van 't Veer C, Mann KG. Regulation of tissue factor initiated thrombin generation by the stoichiometric inhibitors tissue factor pathway inhibitor, antithrombin-III, and heparin cofactor-II. J Biol Chem. 1997; 272: 4367-77.

[176]   Pitlick FA. Concanavalin A inhibits tissue factor coagulant activity. J Clin Invest. 1975; 55: 175-9.

[177]   Paborsky LR, Harris RJ. Post-translational modifications of recombinant human tissue factor. Thromb Res. 1990; 60: 367-76.

[178]   Rickles FR, Contrino J, Kreutzer DL. Reply to "Tissue factor expression in normal and abnormal mammary gland". Nat Med. 1996; 2: 491-2.

[179]   Waxman E, Ross JB, Laue TM, Guha A, Thiruvikraman SV, Lin TC, Konigsberg WH, Nemerson Y. Tissue factor and its extracellular soluble domain: the relationship between intermolecular association with factor VIIa and enzymatic activity of the complex. Biochemistry. 1992; 31: 3998-4003.

[180]   Stone MJ, Ruf W, Miles DJ, Edgington TS, Wright PE. Recombinant soluble human tissue factor secreted by Saccharomyces cerevisiae and refolded from Escherichia coli inclusion bodies: glycosylation of mutants, activity and physical characterization. Biochem J. 1995; 310 (Pt 2): 605-14.

[181]   Shands JW, Jr. Macrophage factor X activator formation: metabolic requirements for synthesis of components. Blood. 1985; 65: 169-75.

[182]   Bona R, Lee E, Rickles F. Tissue factor apoprotein: intracellular transport and expression in shed membrane vesicles. Thromb Res. 1987; 48: 487-500.

[183]   Krudysz-Amblo J, Jennings ME, 2nd, Matthews DE, Mann KG, Butenas S. Differences in the fractional abundances of carbohydrates of natural and recombinant human tissue factor. Biochim Biophys Acta. 2011; 1810: 398-405.

[184]   Zioncheck TF, Roy S, Vehar GA. The cytoplasmic domain of tissue factor is phosphorylated by a protein kinase C-dependent mechanism. J Biol Chem. 1992; 267: 3561-4.

[185]   Mody RS, Carson SD. Tissue factor cytoplasmic domain peptide is multiply phosphorylated in vitro. Biochemistry. 1997; 36: 7869-75.

[186]   Egorina EM, Sovershaev MA, Osterud B. Regulation of tissue factor procoagulant activity by post-translational modifications. Thromb Res. 2008; 122: 831-7.

[187]   Rehemtulla A, Ruf W, Edgington TS. The integrity of the cysteine 186-cysteine 209 bond of the second disulfide loop of tissue factor is required for binding of factor VII. J Biol Chem. 1991; 266: 10294-9.

[188]   Krudysz-Amblo J, Jennings ME, 2nd, Knight T, Matthews DE, Mann KG, Butenas S. Disulfide reduction abolishes tissue factor cofactor function. Biochim Biophys Acta. 2013; 1830: 3489-96.

[189]   van den Hengel LG, Kocaturk B, Reitsma PH, Ruf W, Versteeg HH. Complete abolishment of coagulant activity in monomeric disulfide-deficient tissue factor. Blood. 2011; 118: 3446-8.

[190]   Chen VM, Ahamed J, Versteeg HH, Berndt MC, Ruf W, Hogg PJ. Evidence for activation of tissue factor by an allosteric disulfide bond. Biochemistry. 2006; 45: 12020-8.

[191]   Schmidt B, Ho L, Hogg PJ. Allosteric disulfide bonds. Biochemistry. 2006; 45: 7429-33.

[192]   Ruf W, Versteeg HH. Tissue factor mutated at the allosteric Cys186-Cys209 disulfide bond is severely impaired in decrypted procoagulant activity. Blood. 2010; 116: 500-1; author reply 2-3.

[193]   Ahamed J, Versteeg HH, Kerver M, Chen VM, Mueller BM, Hogg PJ, Ruf W. Disulfide isomerization switches tissue factor from coagulation to cell signaling. Proc Natl Acad Sci U S A. 2006; 103: 13932-7.

[194]   Reinhardt C, von Bruhl ML, Manukyan D, Grahl L, Lorenz M, Altmann B, Dlugai S, Hess S, Konrad I, Orschiedt L, Mackman N, Ruddock L, Massberg S, Engelmann B. Protein disulfide isomerase acts as an injury response signal that enhances fibrin generation via tissue factor activation. J Clin Invest. 2008; 118: 1110-22.

[195]   Pendurthi UR, Ghosh S, Mandal SK, Rao LV. Tissue factor activation: is disulfide bond switching a regulatory mechanism? Blood. 2007; 110: 3900-8.

[196]   Kothari H, Sen P, Pendurthi UR, Rao LV. Bovine protein disulfide isomerase-enhanced tissue factor coagulant function: is phospholipid contaminant in it the real culprit? Blood. 2008; 111: 3295-6.

[197]   Popescu NI, Lupu C, Lupu F. Role of PDI in regulating tissue factor: FVIIa activity. Thromb Res. 2010; 125 Suppl 1: S38-41.

[198]   Morrissey JH. Tissue factor: an enzyme cofactor and a true receptor. Thromb Haemost. 2001; 86: 66-74.

[199]   Owens AP, 3rd, Mackman N. Tissue factor and thrombosis: The clot starts here. Thromb Haemost. 2010; 104: 432-9.

[200]   Davizon P, Munday AD, Lopez JA. Tissue factor, lipid rafts, and microparticles. Semin Thromb Hemost. 2010; 36: 857-64.

[201]   Trappenburg MC, van Schilfgaarde M, Marchetti M, Spronk HM, ten Cate H, Leyte A, Terpstra WE, Falanga A. Elevated procoagulant microparticles expressing endothelial and platelet markers in essential thrombocythemia. Haematologica. 2009; 94: 911-8.

[202]   Burnier L, Fontana P, Kwak BR, Angelillo-Scherrer A. Cell-derived microparticles in haemostasis and vascular medicine. Thromb Haemost. 2009; 101: 439-51.

[203]   Blann A, Shantsila E, Shantsila A. Microparticles and arterial disease. Semin Thromb Hemost. 2009; 35: 488-96.

[204]   Himber J, Wohlgensinger C, Roux S, Damico LA, Fallon JT, Kirchhofer D, Nemerson Y, Riederer MA. Inhibition of tissue factor limits the growth of venous thrombus in the rabbit. J Thromb Haemost. 2003; 1: 889-95.

[205]   Roque M, Reis ED, Fuster V, Padurean A, Fallon JT, Taubman MB, Chesebro JH, Badimon JJ. Inhibition of tissue factor reduces thrombus formation and intimal hyperplasia after porcine coronary angioplasty. J Am Coll Cardiol. 2000; 36: 2303-10.

[206]   Suleymanov OD, Szalony JA, Salyers AK, LaChance RM, Parlow JJ, South MS, Wood RS, Nicholson NS. Pharmacological interruption of acute thrombus formation with minimal hemorrhagic

complications by a small molecule tissue factor/factor VIIa inhibitor: comparison to factor Xa and thrombin inhibition in a nonhuman primate thrombosis model. J Pharmacol Exp Ther. 2003; 306: 1115-21.

[207] Young WB, Mordenti J, Torkelson S, Shrader WD, Kolesnikov A, Rai R, Liu L, Hu H, Leahy EM, Green MJ, Sprengeler PA, Katz BA, Yu C, Janc JW, Elrod KC, Marzec UM, Hanson SR. Factor VIIa inhibitors: chemical optimization, preclinical pharmacokinetics, pharmacodynamics, and efficacy in an arterial baboon thrombosis model. Bioorg Med Chem Lett. 2006; 16: 2037-41.

[208] Hatakeyama K, Asada Y, Marutsuka K, Sato Y, Kamikubo Y, Sumiyoshi A. Localization and activity of tissue factor in human aortic atherosclerotic lesions. Atherosclerosis. 1997; 133: 213-9.

[209] Wilcox JN, Smith KM, Schwartz SM, Gordon D. Localization of tissue factor in the normal vessel wall and in the atherosclerotic plaque. Proc Natl Acad Sci U S A. 1989; 86: 2839-43.

[210] Ross R. Atherosclerosis--an inflammatory disease. N Engl J Med. 1999; 340: 115-26.

[211] Ott I, Michaelis C, Schuermann M, Steppich B, Seitz I, Dewerchin M, Zohlnhofer D, Wessely R, Rudelius M, Schomig A, Carmeliet P. Vascular remodeling in mice lacking the cytoplasmic domain of tissue factor. Circ Res. 2005; 97: 293-8.

[212] George FD. Microparticles in vascular diseases. Thromb Res. 2008; 122 Suppl 1: S55-9.

[213] Ettelaie C, Li C, Collier ME, Pradier A, Frentzou GA, Wood CG, Chetter IC, McCollum PT, Bruckdorfer KR, James NJ. Differential functions of tissue factor in the trans-activation of cellular signalling pathways. Atherosclerosis. 2007; 194: 88-101.

[214] Ryden L, Grabau D, Schaffner F, Jonsson PE, Ruf W, Belting M. Evidence for tissue factor phosphorylation and its correlation with protease-activated receptor expression and the prognosis of primary breast cancer. Int J Cancer. 2010; 126: 2330-40.

[215] Schaffner F, Ruf W. Tissue factor and PAR2 signaling in the tumor microenvironment. Arterioscler Thromb Vasc Biol. 2009; 29: 1999-2004.

[216] Vidwan P, Pathak A, Sheth S, Huang J, Monroe DM, Stouffer GA. Activation of protease-activated receptors 3 and 4 accelerates tissue factor-induced thrombin generation on the surface of vascular smooth muscle cells. Arterioscler Thromb Vasc Biol. 2010; 30: 2587-96.

[217] Demetz G, Seitz I, Stein A, Steppich B, Groha P, Brandl R, Schomig A, Ott I. Tissue Factor-Factor VIIa complex induces cytokine expression in coronary artery smooth muscle cells. Atherosclerosis. 2010; 212: 466-71.

[218] So AK, Varisco PA, Kemkes-Matthes B, Herkenne-Morard C, Chobaz-Peclat V, Gerster JC, Busso N. Arthritis is linked to local and systemic activation of coagulation and fibrinolysis pathways. J Thromb Haemost. 2003; 1: 2510-5.

[219] Levi M, ten Cate H, Bauer KA, van der Poll T, Edgington TS, Buller HR, van Deventer SJ, Hack CE, ten Cate JW, Rosenberg RD. Inhibition of endotoxin-induced activation of coagulation and fibrinolysis by pentoxifylline or by a monoclonal anti-tissue factor antibody in chimpanzees. J Clin Invest. 1994; 93: 114-20.

[220] Chu AJ. Tissue factor mediates inflammation. Arch Biochem Biophys. 2005; 440: 123-32.

[221] Koga H, Sugiyama S, Kugiyama K, Watanabe K, Fukushima H, Tanaka T, Sakamoto T, Yoshimura M, Jinnouchi H, Ogawa H. Elevated levels of VE-cadherin-positive endothelial microparticles in patients with type 2 diabetes mellitus and coronary artery disease. J Am Coll Cardiol. 2005; 45: 1622-30.

[222] Cuccuini W, Poitevin S, Poitevin G, Dignat-George F, Cornillet-Lefebvre P, Sabatier F, Nguyen P. Tissue factor up-regulation in proinflammatory conditions confers thrombin generation capacity to endothelial colony-forming cells without influencing non-coagulant properties in vitro. J Thromb Haemost. 2010; 8: 2042-52.

[223] Kasthuri RS, Taubman MB, Mackman N. Role of tissue factor in cancer. J Clin Oncol. 2009; 27: 4834-8.

[224] White RH, Chew H, Wun T. Targeting patients for anticoagulant prophylaxis trials in patients with cancer: who is at highest risk? Thromb Res. 2007; 120 Suppl 2: S29-40.

[225] Nash GF, Walsh DC, Kakkar AK. The role of the coagulation system in tumour angiogenesis. Lancet Oncol. 2001; 2: 608-13.

[226] Belting M, Ahamed J, Ruf W. Signaling of the tissue factor coagulation pathway in angiogenesis and cancer. Arterioscler Thromb Vasc Biol. 2005; 25: 1545-50.

[227]   Abe K, Shoji M, Chen J, Bierhaus A, Danave I, Micko C, Casper K, Dillehay DL, Nawroth PP, Rickles FR. Regulation of vascular endothelial growth factor production and angiogenesis by the cytoplasmic tail of tissue factor. Proc Natl Acad Sci U S A. 1999; 96: 8663-8.

[228]   Takano S, Tsuboi K, Tomono Y, Mitsui Y, Nose T. Tissue factor, osteopontin, alphavbeta3 integrin expression in microvasculature of gliomas associated with vascular endothelial growth factor expression. Br J Cancer. 2000; 82: 1967-73.

[229]   Mueller BM, Reisfeld RA, Edgington TS, Ruf W. Expression of tissue factor by melanoma cells promotes efficient hematogenous metastasis. Proc Natl Acad Sci U S A. 1992; 89: 11832-6.

[230]   Ueno T, Toi M, Koike M, Nakamura S, Tominaga T. Tissue factor expression in breast cancer tissues: its correlation with prognosis and plasma concentration. Br J Cancer. 2000; 83: 164-70.

[231]   Lwaleed BA, Francis JL, Chisholm M. Urinary tissue factor levels in patients with bladder and prostate cancer. Eur J Surg Oncol. 2000; 26: 44-9.

[232]   Seto S, Onodera H, Kaido T, Yoshikawa A, Ishigami S, Arii S, Imamura M. Tissue factor expression in human colorectal carcinoma: correlation with hepatic metastasis and impact on prognosis. Cancer. 2000; 88: 295-301.

[233]   Yu JL, May L, Lhotak V, Shahrzad S, Shirasawa S, Weitz JI, Coomber BL, Mackman N, Rak JW. Oncogenic events regulate tissue factor expression in colorectal cancer cells: implications for tumor progression and angiogenesis. Blood. 2005; 105: 1734-41.

58

CHAPTER 3

Hemostasis: General Principles

Melda Comert, Fahri Sahin and Guray Saydam[*]

Ege University Hospital, Department of Hematology, Bornova, Izmir, Turkey

Abstract: Hemostasis is the physiological process of clot formation in a delicate balance in the human body after a vessel injury. That process represents primary and secondary haemostasis that includes platelets, coagulation proteins and finally terminates with fibrinolysis to prevent widespread clot formation.

Keywords: Coagulation cascade, endotelium, fibrin, fibrinolysis, hemostasis, plasminogen, platelets, primary hemostasis, secondary hemostasis, subendothelial matrix, tissue factor, vonWillebrand factor.

INTRODUCTION

Hemostasis defines the perfect physiological balance between coagulation and fibrinolysis for avoidance of pathological bleeding or thrombosis. The rapid transformation of blood within seconds into a thrombus at the localized site of tissue injury without any harmful effect on normal blood flow is administered by dynamic interactions of four components: the vessel wall, platelets, the coagulation proteins and fibrinolysis [1].

The complexity of hemostatic system has been increasingly evaluated in few decades. Vessel wall is surfaced by endotelium which forms a continuous monolayer between blood and tissue for maintaining nonthrombotic surface for blood fluidity. Also endotelium keeps platelets in inactive status, minimizes the thrombin formation and provides deposition of fibrin in the microvasculature [2]. Endotelium is critical for initiating the inflammatory response. After the blood vessel damage, highly reactive subendothelial matrix components are exposed to the circulation that activate the main processes of hemostasis to initiate formation of a hemostatic plug, composed primarily of platelets and fibrin mesh simultaneously.

One of the steps of hemostasis referred to primary hemostasis includes platelet attachement, spreading, secretion, aggregation and platelet plug formation

---

*Corresponding author Guray Saydam: Ege University Hospital, Department of Hematology, 35100 Bornova, Izmir, Turkey; E-mail: guray.saydam@ege.edu.tr

Ertugrul Ercan and Gulfem Ece (Eds.)

initiated by adhesive proteins, collagen and thrombin to arrest bleeding rapidly [3]. Secondary hemostasis refers to the deposition of insoluble fibrin mesh which is generated by the proteolytic coagulation cascade [1]. It is triggered by pro-coagulant factors like fibrinogen, factor V, von Willebrand factor (vWF) and by tissue factor (TF) as a critical component of vascular elements. The fibrin mesh binds the platelets and contributes to their attachment to the vessel defect, mediated by binding the platelet receptor glycoproteins and by interactions with other adhesive proteins such as thrombospondin, fibronectin and vitronectin [4].

After the stabilization of the hemostatic plug, local reparative processes restore normal vascular structure and the fibrinolytic system reconstitutes clearence of the vascular lumen [2]. This chapter focuses on the general principles of hemostasis and thrombosis regulation.

VASCULAR ENDOTHELIUM

The monolayer of cells that surface the interior of blood vessels, known as the endothelium, plays a complex role in vascular biology [5]. Endothelial cells (ECs) cover the entire vasculature of human body comprised of blood and lymphatic vessels with a large surface and it is the largest organ in the body composed of 1-6 x 10^{13} cells, 720 g and 4000 to 7000 m^2 surface area in an adult person [6-7]. Most of these cells are microvascular endothelial cells, and cover the surface of capillaries [8]. The role of endothelial injury in hemostasis and thrombosis has been known for 4 decades. But recent developments, such as in risk factors and inflammation have placed endothelium at the centre of the pathogenesis of atherosclerosis [7]. One of the most important role of vascular endothelium is to provide a thromboresistant layer. Endothelial protection mechanisms from thrombosis depends on the comprising glycocalyx that produces heparan- and dermatan-sulfate molecules to activate heparin cofactor II and antithrombin (AT), expression of tissue factor pathway inhibitor (TFPI) that limits the activity of the extrinsic pathway, the activation of the protein C /protein S system that downregulates the intrinsic coagulation route and the expression of tissue plasminogen activator (tPA) and urokinase for dissolution of microthrombi [9, 10]. Additionally, the endothelium has anti-oxidant and anti-inflammatory roles that regulates leukocyte adhesion and migration, smooth muscle proliferation and migration [11, 12].

Vasoconstriction is an important initial response when the vessel is damaged. Extracellular matrix (ECM) proteins (Glycoprotein (GP)Ib, GPVI, VWF, TF, plasminogen activator inhibitor type 1 (PAI-1), laminin, fibronectin, thrombospondin, cytokines, growth factors, chemokines, leukocyte, and platelet adhesion molecules (vascular cell adhesion molecule [VCAM], intercellular adhesion molecule [ICAM]) and some integrins that synthesized and deposited by ECs are exposed after the injury to serve as ligands for different platelet surface receptors [10]. Following the exposure, primary hemostasis is triggered.

PRIMARY HEMOSTASIS

Primary hemostasis refers to the early stages of hemostasis and platelets have a critical role in this process. Platelets are small anucleated cell fragments that follow the entirety of the vascular system and most platelets never firm adhesion and are finally cleared by macrophages in spleen and liver. Only in response to traumatic injury or pathological modification of the endothelium like atherosclerosis [13], platelets rapidly moved up against exposed matrix, adhere, activated, and bind further platelets to form a thrombus preventing further bleeding but limited in size [14] (Fig. **1**).

First step is the platelet and vessel wall interaction that called "adhesion". VWF synthesized by endothelium and secreted into both plasma and the ECM, binds specifically to sites on exposed collagen and is stretched by the shear stress of the flowing blood to expose binding sites on the A1 domains for adhesive platelet receptor complex GPIb (part of GPIb-IX-V complex) on platelets. Following platelet contact with the VWF-coated subendothelial matrix, GPIb binds to VWF at the contact site [13]. It draws out the patch of bound GPIb together with membrane and associated cytoskeleton to form an elongated strong bound to bring the platelet to a standstill in contact with the subendothelium [15].

Second step is platelet activation. The major signalling receptor involved in this step is thought to be GPVI *via* binding to specific GPO (glycine-proline-hydroxyproline) sites on exposed collagens to activate platelets [16]. In this process two glycoproteins are important: $\alpha2\beta1$ and $\alpha IIb\beta3$ that are activated by GPVI interaction with collagen and releasing the content of α- and dense granules. Integrins $\alpha IIb\beta3$ and $\alpha2\beta1$ are normally present on the platelet surface in an inactive form, but platelet activation induces a conformational transition in these receptors that exposes ligand binding sites [17]. $\alpha IIb\beta3$ is the most important receptor as it is present at the highest density on the platelet surface [18]. Adenosine diphosphate (ADP) and serotonin secretion from dense granules and Thromboxan A2 (TxA2) that released by stimulated platelets, activates further platelets by the Gq-and G12/13-coupled thromboxane-prostanoid receptors TPα and TPβ thereby promoting plug formation.

Another critical mechanism of platelet activation that links secondary hemostasis to platelet function is activation by the terminal serine protease of the coagulation cascade; thrombin. Thrombin cleaves 2 protease activated receptors (PARs) on human platelets, PAR1 and PAR4. These receptors cleavage by thrombin exposes a new N-terminus that serves as a tethered ligand to activate the receptor [1, 18] and initiate cell-signaling pathways that results in platelet granule secretion, integrin activation, and platelet cytoskeleton remodeling [19].

Platelet adhesion and activation is followed by the third step called "aggregation" leading to the formation of a fibrinogen-rich thrombus at the site of injury. This step is mediated by agonist induced activation of integrin αIIbβ3 that changes its conformation from a resting to an activated conformation allowing interaction with fibrinogen. Due to the symmetric nature of fibrinogen, platelets are bridged and platelet aggregates are formed. VWF and fibronectin contributes to the formation of stable platelet aggregates and stability of the thrombus is mediated by adhesion and signaling receptors [20] and deposition of insoluble fibrin generated by the coagulation cascade as described below.

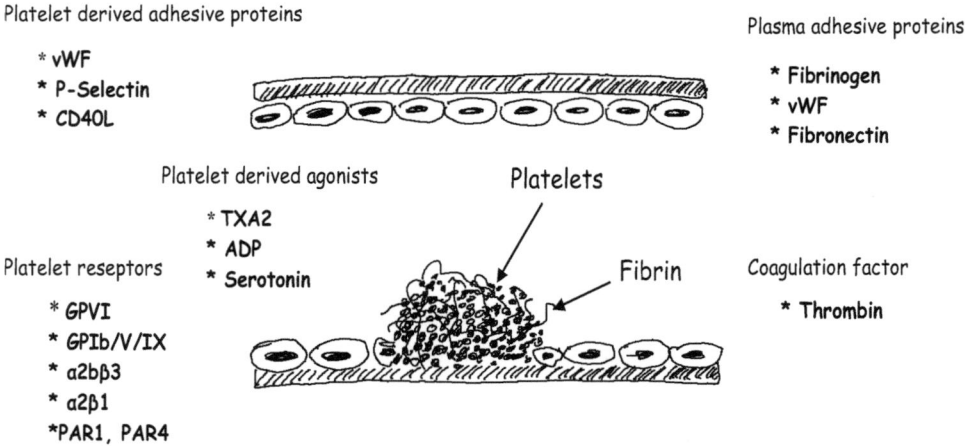

Figure 1: Primary hemostasis started by platelet adhesion and followed by platelet activation and aggregation. Primary hemostasis at the area of damage is operated by platelet receptors, platelet-derived agonists, platelet derived adhesive proteins, and plasma-derived adhesive proteins. Coagulation cascade is actively involved after this step to accumulate fibrin around platelet plug.

SECONDARY HEMOSTASIS

First coagulation model was composed by Morawitz in 1905 [21]. Concept of secondary hemostasis revised in recent years. This process consists of thrombin that generated by vascular damage-induced exposure of subendothelial TF [22]. In healthy blood vessels, this cascade is not activated, and presence of thrombomodulin and heparan sulfate proteoglycans on vascular endothelium prevent its activation. When the vascular damage occurs, blood is exposed to extravascular tissues, which are rich in TF also known as thromboplastin serving as a coagulation initiator. Association of plasma factor VII with activated Factor VII (FVII/VIIa) is the ligand for TF. The binding of FVII/VIIa to newly exposed TF at the site of damage provides autocatalytic conversion of FVII to FVIIa [2]. The complex of TF and factor VIIa indirectly activates factor X and factor IX. This activation pathway was historically termed as "extrinsic pathway". Factor IXa activates factor X, in conjunction with its cofactor factor VIIIa. Factor Xa acivates prohrombin to constitute thrombin with the presence of cofactor factor Va [1].

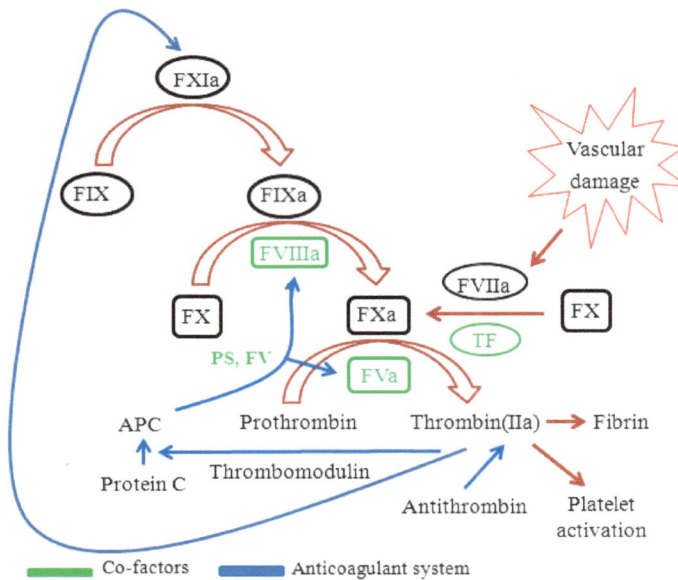

Figure 2: Secondary hemostasis; the coagulation cascade and the anticoagulant system [1, 25]. F: Factor, PS: Protein S, APC: Active protein C.

Thrombin activates platelets *via* cleavage of PAR1 and PAR4 and factor XI, which then activates factor IX, and thrombin activates cofactors VIII and V. This was historically called the "intrinsic pathway" [23].

After the occlution of the damaged vessel by hemostatic clot, down-regulation of the coagulation cascade must be activated to prevent uncontrolled, widespread clot formation. This procces include antithrombins (majorly antithrombin and heparin co-factor II) which inhibit the serine proteases of the coagulation system; and the protein C system which neutralizes activated coagulation co-factors. Antithrombin inhibits factors IXa, Xa and thrombin [24]. Protein C has a high homology to the vitamin K-dependent procoagulant factor. APC cleaves and inactivates the procoagulant cofactors VIIIa and Va in presence of cofactors protein S and a vitamin K-dependent protein. Besides this, factor V provides anticoagulant function as a cofactor for APC/protein S in the inactivation of factor VIIIa and factor Va [25].

FIBRINOLYSIS

Finally, the process of clot dissolution that functions as both a clot limiting mechanism and as a process of repair known as fibrinolysis, initiate [25]. The fibrinolytic system is composed primarily of three serine proteases; plasminogen, proteases tissue-type plasminogen activator (tPA) and urokinase-type plasminogen activator (uPA) that are present as zymogens [26]. Plasminogen is the key player in fibrinolysis and is generates plasmin by tPA and uPA. Plasmin cleaves and breaks down fibrin by hydrolysing arginine and lysine bonds, resulting in proteolysis of its major substrates, fibrinogen and fibrin but also factors V, VIII and XIII [25]. tPA activates plasminogen and uPA activates plasminogen in the presence of the uPA receptor on the surface of a fbrin clot. (Fig. **3**)

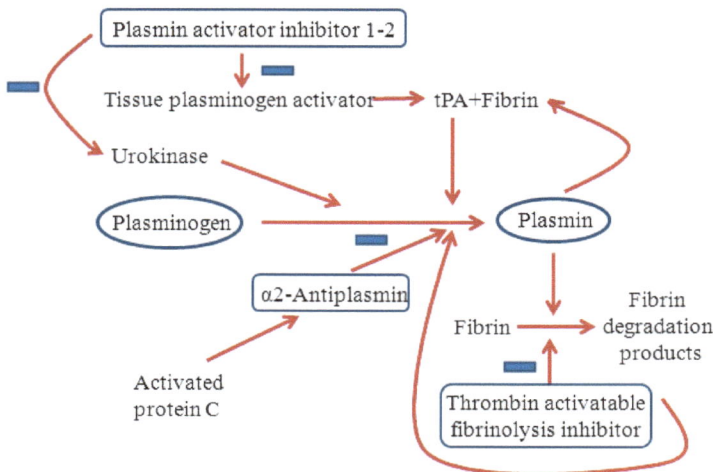

Figure 3: Fibrinolytic system.

Excessive fibrinolysis resulting in fibrinogen consumption and haemorrhage is regulated by specific plasminogen activator inhibitors (PAIs). There are 3 types of PAIs described that α2-Antiplasmin and PAI-1 and PAI-2. α2-Antiplasmin inhibits plasmin and PAI-1 and PAI-2 inhibit tPA and uPA [27, 28]. Further control of fibrinolysis occurs *via* thrombin activatable fibrinolysis inhibitor (TAFI) that provides a direct moleculer link between the coagulation cascade and fibrinolytic system [29].

ACKNOWLEDGEMENTS

Declared none.

CONFLICT OF INTEREST

The authors confirm that this chapter contents have no conflict of interest.

REFERENCES

[1]   Gale AJ Current Understanding of Hemostasis. Toxicol Pathol 2011; 39(1): 273-280.
[2]   Schafer AI. Overview of Hemostasis and Fibrinolysis. In: New Therapeutic Agents in Thrombosis and Thrombolysis. 3rd edition, edt Jane E. Freedman and Joseph Loscalzo. Healthcare, New York, 1-8.
[3]   Hoffman, ACS and Plow EF. The molecular basis of Platelet Function. In Hematology Basic Principles and Practice (R. Hoffman, E. J. Benz, S. J. Shattil, B. Furie, L. E. Silberstein, and P. McGlave, eds.) 2009, 5th ed., pp. 1781-1791. Churchill Livingstone, New York.
[4]   Rasche H. Haemostasis and thrombosis: an overview. European Heart Journal 2001; 3(Q): 3-7.
[5]   Liao JK. Linking endothelial dysfunction with endothelial cell activation. The Journal of Clinical Investigation 2013; 123(2): 540-541.
[6]   van Hinsbergh VWM. Endothelium-role in regulation of coagulation and inflammation. Semin Immunopathol 2012; 34: 93-106.
[7]   Gimbrone MA *et al*. 1986, Vascular endothelium: nature's blood container. In: Vascular endothelium in hemostasis and thrombosis. Churchill Livingstone, New York, pp 1-13.
[8]   Wolinsky HA proposal linking clearance of circulating lipoproteins to tissue metabolic-activity as a basis for understanding atherogenesis. Circ Res 1980; 47: 301-311.
[9]   Becker BF, Heindl B, Kupatt C, Zahler S. Endothelial function and hemostasis. Z Kardiol 2000; 89: 160-167.
[10]   Kleinegris MC, ten Cate-Hoek AJ, ten Cate H. Coagulation and the vessel wall in thrombosis and atherosclerosis. Polskie archiwum medycyny wewnętrznej 2012; 122(11): 557-566.
[11]   Ramcharan KS, Lip GYH, Stonelake PS, Blann AD. The endotheliome: A new concept in vascular biology. Thromb Res 2011; 128(1): 1-7.
[12]   Thomas SR, Witting PK, Drummond GR. Redox control of endothelial function and dysfunction: molecular mechanisms and therapeutic opportunities. Antioxid Redox Signal 2008; 10: 1713-1765.
[13]   Stegner D, Nieswandt B. Platelet receptor signaling in thrombus formation. J Mol Med 2011; 89: 109-121.
[14]   Clemetson K. J. Platelets and Primary Haemostasis. Thrombosis Research 2012; 129: 220-224.
[15]   Dopheide SM, Maxwell MJ, Jackson SP. Shear-dependent tether formation during platelet translocation on von Willebrand factor. Blood 2002; 99: 159-67.
[16]   Clemetson JM, Polgar J, Magnenat E, Wells TN, Clemetson KJ. The platelet collagen receptor glycoprotein VI is a member of the immunoglobulin superfamily closely related to FcαR and the natural killer receptors. J Biol Chem 1999; 274: 29019-29024.

[17]   Xiao T, Takagi J, Coller BS, Wang JH, Springer TA. Structural basis for allostery in integrins and binding to fibrinogenmimetic therapeutics. Nature 2004; 432: 59-67.

[18]   Vu TK, Hung DT, Wheaton VI, Coughlin SR. Molecular cloning of a functional thrombin receptor reveals a novel proteolytic mechanism of receptor activation. Cell 1991; 64: 1057-1068.

[19]   Brass LF. The molecular basis for platelet activation. In Hematology Basic Principles and Practice (R. Hoffman, E. J. Benz, S. J. Shattil, B. Furie, L. E. Silberstein, and P. McGlave, eds.), 3rd ed., pp. 1753-70. Churchill Livingstone, New York.

[20]   Brass LF, Zhu L, Stalker TJ. Minding the gaps to promote thrombus growth and stability. J Clin Invest 2005; 115: 3385-3392.

[21]   Riddel JP Jr, Aouizerat BE, Miaskowski C, Lillicrap DP. Theories of blood coagulation. J Pediatr Oncol Nurs 2007; 24: 123-131.

[22]   Versteeg HH, Heemskerk JWM, Levi M, Reitsma PH. New Fundamentals in hemostasis. Physiol Rev 2013; 93: 327-358.

[23]   Bouma BN, von dem Borne PA, Meijers JC. Factor XI and protection of the fibrin clot against lysis—a role for the intrinsic pathway of coagulation in fibrinolysis. Thromb Haemost 1998; 80: 24-27.

[24]   Austin KS. Haemostasis. Medicine 2008; 37(3): 133-136.

[25]   Cramer TJ, Griffin JH, Gale, AJ. Factor V Is an anticoagulant cofactor for activated protein C during inactivation of factor Va. Pathophysiol Haemost Thromb 2010; 37: 17-23.

[26]   Lijnen HR, Collen, D. Molecular and cellular basis of fibrinolysis. In Hematology Basic Principles and Practice (R. Hoffman, E. J. Benz, S. J. Shattil, B. Furie, L. E. Silberstein, and P. McGlave, eds.), 2000, 3rd ed., pp. 1804-14. Churchill Livingstone, New York.

[27]   Zorio E, Gilabert-Estellés J, España F, *et al.* Fibrinolysis: the key to new pathogenetic mechanisms. Curr Med Chem. 2008; 15(9): 923-929.

[28]   Rau, JC, Beaulieu LM, Huntington JA, Church FC. Serpins in thrombosis, hemostasis and fibrinolysis. J Thromb Haemost 2007; 5(1): 102-115.

[29]   Hirsch E, Katanaev VL, Garlanda C, *et al.* Central role for Gprotein-coupled phosphoinositide 3-kinase gamma in inflammation. Science 2000; 287: 1049-1053.

Recurrent Thromboembolism

Melda Comert, Guray Saydam and Fahri Sahin[*]

Ege University Hospital, Department of Hematology, Bornova, Izmir, Turkey

Abstract: Venous thromboembolism (VTE) is a common and preventable disorder which mostly manifests as deep-vein thrombosis of the legs. The incidence of VTE is 1 to 2 cases per 1000 persons in developed countries. After the first episode of VTE risk of recurrence increases in these patients, the cumulative rate of recurrence is about 25% and 30% at 5 years and 10 years respectively. Independent predictors of late recurrence include increasing patient age and body mass index, leg paresis, active cancer and other persistent VTE risk factors such as idiopathic VTE, antiphospholipid antibody syndrome, antithrombin, protein C or protein S deficiency, hyperhomocysteinemia and a persistently increased plasma fibrin D-dimer. The most important point during evaluation of VTE is not to forget that it is a multi-factorial status and can be caused by interaction between the systems which should be investigated carefully.

Keywords: Acquired hypercoagulability, Activated Protein C Resistance, Antiphospholipid Syndrome, anti-thrombin, Clotting, Coagulation, D-dimer, Dysfibrinogenemia, Fibrin, Hyperhomocysteinemia, Inherited hypercoagulability, Platelets, protein C, protein S, Prothrombin gene mutation, recurrence, risk factors, Thrombin, thromboembolism, Thrombophila, thrombosis.

INTODUCTION

VTE is a common and preventable disorder which mostly manifests as deep-vein thrombosis of the legs, or, if embolisation occurs, as pulmonary embolism with high morbidity and mortality. Thrombosis may rarely occur in other veins (cerebral sinus, deep and superficial veins in the arms, retina, and mesentery) [1, 2]. The incidence of VTE is 1 to 2 cases per 1000 persons in developed countries [3, 4] An estimated 200,000 new cases occur in the United States every year, including 94,000 with PE, resulting in an incidence of 23 per 100,000 patients per year-cases. Without treatment, pulmonary embolism is associated with a mortality rate of approximately 30%, causing nearly 50,000 deaths per year. The risk of the disorder rises exponentially with age, from an annual rate of less than 5 per

Corresponding author Fahri Sahin: Ege University Hospital, Department of Hematology, 35100 Bornova, Izmir, Turkey; E-mail: fahri.sahin@ege.edu.tr

Ertugrul Ercan and Gulfem Ece (Eds.)

100,000 children to greater than 400 per 100,000 adults older than 80 years [5]. The overall incidence of a first venous thromboembolism seems to be similar among men and women, [5] but the risk is higher among women of childbearing age than among men in the same age group [6-8]. This difference probably relates to the association of venous thromboembolism with pregnancy or the use of oral contraceptives. By contrast, the risk among older women is substantially lower than that among men in the same age group [6-8]. After the first episode of VTE risk of recurrence increases in these patients, the cumulative rate of recurrence is about 25% at 5 years and 30% at 10 years. The highest incidence of recurrence is in the first 6 months. Independent predictors of late recurrence include increasing patient age and body mass index, leg paresis, active cancer and other persistent VTE risk factors such as idiopathic VTE, antiphospholipid antibody syndrome, antithrombin, protein C or protein S deficiency, hyperhomocysteinemia and a persistently increased plasma fibrin D-dimer [9].

Because of high morbidity, mortality and high recurrence rates a careful evolution and determination of risk factors and effective prophlaxis are important in these patients.

PATHOGENESIS

Venous thrombi are composed of predominantly fibrin and erythrocytes with variable amounts of platelets and leukocytes [10]. In contrast, arterial thrombi are predominantly composed of platelets with fibrin [11]. The initial fibrin nidus will grow by apposition leading to more and more occlusion of venous segments.

Thrombosis implies one or more of three essential states, known as Virchow's triad: (1) local vessel or tissue injury, (2) circulatory stasis, and (3) activation of blood coagulability (inherited or acquired hypercoagulable states). At least 2 of these 3 states, especially circulatuar stasis, in combination are caused venous thrombosis experimentally and in clinical practice.

The development of venous thrombosis is greatly influenced by altered blood flow conditions such as immobility (after especially orthopedic surgery, paraplegic patients), venous obstruction (pelvic tumors), increased venous pressure (increased central venous pressure in heart failure, pregnancy), venous dilation (affect of estrogen in pregnancy, in patients taken estrogen as a treatment, bedridden patients) and increased blood viscosity (polistemia, hipergamaglobulinemia, disproteinemias).

Vessel wall damage in the development of venous thrombosis is at present uncertain, unless venous distension, indeed leads to endothelial damage. This endotelial damage occurs by trauma or endotoxin inflamatory cytokines like IL1, TNF, thrombin. After the endotelial damage, tissue factor will be released, platelets will adhere and aggregate, and the coagulation cascade of clotting will be activated.

Circulatory stasis may contribute to thrombogenesis because of stagnation of the blood with associated local hypoxia, which stimulates endothelial cell release of an activator of blood coagulation.

Hypercoagulability occurs by inherited or acquired changes in balance of coagulation and fibrinolytic factors and their inhibitors which serve to maintain blood fluidity and hemostasis.

Arterial thrombosis generally occurs as a complication of atherosclerosis. Atherosclerosis is the most common underlying cause of coronary heart disease, cerebrovascular disease, and peripheral arterial disease.

RISK FACTORS FOR VTE

It has been speculated that the development of VTE results from interactions between multiple genetic and environmental risk factors [12, 13]. The history in a patient with thrombosis should comprise age at the first thrombotic event, location of the thrombosis and presence of risk factors. A previous venous thromboembolism is the most important risk factor for predicting recurrence of the condition. Major risk factors for venous thromboembolism are summarized in Table **1**.

Table 1: Major risk factors for venous thromboembolism

Acquired	Hereditary
• Surgery (especially orthopedic)	• Prothrombin gene mutation
• Trauma	• Protein C or S deficiency
• Previous thromboembolism	• Antithrombin deficiency
• Prolonged immobility and paralysis	• Hyperhomocysteinemia
• Malignancy	• Elevated levels of factor VIII
• Congestive heart failure	• Dysfibrinogenemia
• Obesity	
• Advanced age (>40)	
• Pregnancy and puerperium	
• Varicose veins	
• Hyperhomocysteinemia	

• Antiphospholipid antibody syndrome	
• Drugs (Tamoxifen, thalidomide, lenalidomide, Oral contraceptives, hormone replacement therapy)	
• Presence of central venous catheter	
• Myeloproliferative disorders	
• İnflammatory bowel disease	
• Nephrotic syndrome	

These risk factors are classified either as reversibl/transient and irreversibl/persistent risk factors. Transient risk factors such as surgery, trauma, immobilisation, confined to bed, pregnancy, drugs, lengthy travel are associated with a lower risk of reccurrence after anticoagulant therapy is discontinued. Patients with a transient risk provoking risk factor do not require further testing because of low risk of recurrence, conversely patients with idiopathic VTE, are at high risk of recurrence. Prandoni and *et al.*, were followed 1626 patients with a first episode of proximal DVT/PE for up to 10 years. The cumulative incidence rates of recurrent VTE were 15% at 1 year, 40.8% after 5 years and 52.6% after 10 years in patients with idiopathic VTE, compared with 6.6% at 1 year, 16.1% after 5 years and 22.5% after 10 years in patients with a provoked event [14].

ANTI-THROMBIN III DEFICIENCY

Antithrombin (AT) functions as a potent natural anticoagulant and serine protease inhibitor that inactivates many enzymes in the coagulation cascade. Herediter deficiency or a range of secondar disorders such as liver dysfunction, sepsis, major surgery like cardiopulmonary bypass, may raise reduced plasma AT levels [15]. Her019ed
HerYou. Hereditery AT III deficiency is a rare disorder that inherited in an autosomal dominant fashion and thus affects both sexes equally and reduces functional AT levels to 40-60% of normal. Patients with hereditary AT deficiency have a ≥50% life time risk of VTE and associated with a three to seven fold higher risk of VTE compared with other thrombophilias [16]. The challenge in managing these patients is preventing potentially life-threatening thrombosis, while minimising the equally significant risk of haemorrhage associated with long-term anticoagulation. Because of this hemorrahage risk, long-term anticoagulation thromboprophlaxis is not recommended to asymptomatic patients. Treatment guidelines recommend short-term thromboprophylaxis with low molecular weight heparin (LMWH) in high-risk clinical settings such as surgery, trauma, management of pregnancy, labour, and delivery. The goal of treatment for patients with hereditary AT deficiency is an initial increase in AT activity to > or

= 120% of normal levels followed by maintenance of AT activity at > or = 80% of normal levels. Plasma-derived AT, heparin, fresh frozen plasma, and human recombinant AT are treatment options for individuals with hereditary AT deficiency [16].

PROTEIN S AND C DEFICIENCY

Protein S, a vitamin K-dependent physiological anticoagulant, acts as a nonenzymatic cofactor to activated protein C in the proteolytic degradation of factor Va and factor VIIIa. Decreased levels or impaired function of protein S leads to decreased degradation of factor Va and factor VIIIa and an increased propensity to venous thrombosis. Acquired protein S deficiency occurs during pregnancy, in association with the use of oral contraceptives and L-asparaginase, DIC and liver diseases.

The prevalence of protein C deficiency has been estimated to about 0.2% to 0.5% of the general population. The clinical presentation of hereditary protein C deficiency is highly variable. Homozygosity and compound heterozygosity have been linked to severe venous thrombotic complications early in the life but there is no association with arterial thrombosis. Heterozygous patients have a moderate form of the disease with 8 to 10 fold relative risk of DVT during adulthood. Patients are rarely symptomatic until early 20s but by the time number of thrombotic events increase. Approximetaly 63% of affected patients develop recurrent venous thrombosis.

ACTIVATED PROTEIN C RESISTANCE (APCR) AND FACTOR V LEIDEN MUTATION

APC is a normal component of blood that contributes to antithrombotic mechanism and prevent thrombosis. Factor V circulates in plasma as an inactive cofactor. Activation by thrombin results in the formation of factor Va which serves as a cofactor in the conversion of prothrombin to thrombin. The molecular basis of the laboratory phenotype of resistance to APC was found to be mutation in the gene codding for coagulation factor V and this gene product called as factor V leiden. There are two causes of APC resistance, genetic and acquired. Heterozygosity for the factor V Leiden mutation accounts for 90% to 95% of cases of APC resistance phenotype. Acquired states such as pregnancy, elevated factor VIII levels, use of oral contraceptives, presence of antiphospholipid antibodies can involve first generation resistance adjustments. The factor V leiden mutation leads to hypercoagulable state for two reasons; 1- increased coagulation: factor Va leiden is inactivated 10 times slower by APC than normal factor Va. 2-

decreased anticoagulation: factor V leiden decreases the anticoagulant activity of activated protein C.

Factor V Leiden is the most common cause of inherited thrombophilia, accounting for 40% - 50% of cases. Between 1% and 8,5% of individuals in Caucasions have been documented to be heterozygosity for factor V leiden. Homozygosity account for about 1% of patients with the factor V leiden mutation. Individuals homozygous for the mutation have a 70 - fold and heterogenous have a 4 - 8 fold enhance relative risk of venous thrombosis.

HYPERHOMOCYSTEINEMIA

Hyperhomocysteinemia is a rare autosomal recessive disease which increases risk of both arterial and venous thrombosis. Increased plasma homocysteine levels can occur due to genetic defects in the enzymes involved in homocysteine metabolism, to nutritional deficiencies in vitamin cofactors folate, vitamin B6, and/or vitamin B12, or to other factors like smoking, renal insufficiency and drugs such as fibrates, nicotinic acid and phenytoin. The most common form of genetic hyperhomocysteinemia results from production of a thermolabile variant of methylene tetrahydrofolate reductase (MTHFR) with reduced enzymatic activity [17]. Moderate hyperhomocysteinemia is an independent risk factor for atherosclerotic vascular disease and recurrent venous thromboembolism. Hyperhomocysteinemia tends to coagulapathy include increased platelet adhesion, activation of coagulation cascade, conversion of LDL to pro-atherogenic form and endotelial injury that leads to vascular inflammation, which in turn may lead to atherogenesis and can result in ischemic injury. Folat and B12 levels should be checked in all patients and in treatment vitamin supplements which include folate, B6 and B12 should be given.

ANTIPHOSPHOLIPID SYNDROME

Antiphospholipid Syndrome (aPLs) is an acquired, autoimmune, hypercoagulable state caused by antibodies against cell-membrane phospholipids associated with both venous and arterial thrombosis. Classification with aPLs requires evidence of both one or more specific, documented clinical events (either a vascular thrombosis and/or adverse obstetric event) and the confirmed presence of a repeated IgG aPL antibodies on two seperate sample at least 6 weeks distinct. aPLs should be considered in the presence of optic neuropathy, thrombocytopenia, pre-eclampsia, recurrent abortus, SLE, SLE-like syndromes and complicated migraine.

The risk of recurrent VTE is significantly increased in patients with the antiphospholipid syndrome (APS), with hazard ratios ranging from 2.3 to 8.5 in the different studies [18, 19]. In APS patients, thrombosis tends to recur in the same vascular system as the original event. For example, these patients generally have venous rather than arterial recurrent thrombotic events after a first VTE. In 3 retrospective studies, recurrent thrombosis (both arterial and venous) occurred in 52% to 69% of APS patients after 5 to 6.4 years of follow-up, regardless of the preventive strategy [20-22].

This disease is treated by aspirin to inhibit platelet activation, and/or warfarin as an anticoagulant to prevent recurrent systemic thrombosis. During pregnancy, low molecular weight heparin and low-dose aspirin are used instead of warfarin because of warfarin's teratogenicity.

CARDIOVASCULAR RISK FACTORS

Studies suggest that age, male sex, black ethnicity, obesity, smoking, diabetes mellitus, a positive family history of myocardial infarction, and low HDL-cholesterol are associated with risk of venous and arterial thrombosis. A recent meta-analysis confirmed that cardiovascular risk factors are associated with an increased risk of VTE and also recurrent VTE. Long-term incidence of cardiovascular disease has been reported to be higher in patients with idiopathic VTE than in patients with secondary events [23]. Doggen *et al.*, repoted that prothrombin gene mutation was associated with an increased risk of acute myocardial infarction when one of the major cardiovascular risk factors was also present [23]. In a retrospective epidemiological study, obesity was found as an independent risk factor of recurrent thromboembolism [24]. In another retrospective study elevated body mass index (BMI$\geq$25) was associated with recurrent VTE in young women. In a case-control study, an elevated plasma lipoprotein a level was an independent risk factor for idiopathic and recurrent VTE [25]. In an Austrian cohort study low HDL levels were associated with recurrent VTE [26]. Conflicting results have been reported for hypertension, dyslipidemia, physical inactivity, smoking and alcohol association with an increased risk of VTE [27]. Increased D-dimer levels were strongly related with occurence of venous thromboembolim [28].

PROTHROMBIN GENE MUTATIONS

Prothrombin is a vitamin K dependent protein and syntheised in the liver. It is the precursor of thrombin in the coagulation cascade, also called factor II.

Prothrombin gene mutation was first described in 1996 [29]. The gene has a mutation at nucleotid 20210 (guanine to adenine transtion) The mutation leads to increase amount of thrombin. Plasma thrombin levels are higher 30% than normals in heterogous carriers. Thrombotic risk in homozygous for prothrombin gen mutation is substantially higher than that in heterozygous carriers.

This mutation is seen about 1-2 % in the Caucasion population. Prevalance rate of Europe is 0,7 to 4.0%, highest prevalance rate reported in Spain [30]. A study of data from investigation of population with a personal and family history of venous thrombosis found that 18% of these population had prothrombin gene mutation and 40% of these mutation positive patients also had factor V leiden mutation. The prothrombin gene mutation independently conferred a 2,8- fold increased risk of venous thrombosis, it is also reported that prothrombin gene mutation is associated with an increased risk for DVT reccurence, if factor V leiden mutation attends to this mutation, the thrombotic risk increases 3 to 5 fold above the risk of a single defect [31].

PCR methods have been used to detect the both G20210 prothrombin gene mutation and factor V leiden in the same reaction. Plasma prothrombin concentration can not be used to screen for the prothrombin gene mutation.

DYSFIBRINOGENEMIAS

Dysfibrinogenemias are a rare cause of thrombophilia, present bleeding diasthesis or recurrent venous or arterial thrombosis or asymptomatic. These defects are manifested by prolongation of thrombin and reptilase times with fibrinogen levels are normal or lower. The prevalence of thrombosis among patients with dysfibrinogenemias is estimated to around 10 to 20 %, especially venous thrombosis of lower extremity have been seen more frequent than arterial or both arterial/venous thrombosis.

The most important point during evaluation of VTE is not to forget that it is a multi-factorial status and can be caused by interaction between the systems which should be investigated carefully.

Thromboembolic events and VTE in the course of acute coonary syndromes (ACS) can be seen as a result of atrial fibrillation which is found in between 6and 21% of cases, either existing previously or developed within 30 days of ACS. Patients with ACS should be treated with oral anti-coagulant (OAC), not only at the time of event, but also after discharging from hospital. Frequently, the same patients with ACS require treatment withtwo oral antiplatelet agents to prevent ACS and both, VTE and stent occlusion. Although, combined OAC therapy and dual antiplatelet therapy (DAPT) relatively increases potential risks for bleeding and creates a therapeutic dilemma. But, it is needed to be clarified how possible to decrease rate of recurrent ACS and VTE without increasing the risk of bleeding. Unfortunately, there is little clinical trial evidence for most effective and safest strategy.

The Atrial Fibrillation Clopidegrol Trial With Irbesartan for Prevention of Vascular Events-Warfarin (ACTIVE W) study revealed that the risk of stroke can be reduced in chronic atrial fibrillation patients by 42% with treatment of warfarin compared to DAPT with ASA and clopidegrol therapy [32]. The only ASA therapy in patientsineligible for other drugs could decrease the risk with the rate of 28%.

The studies with dabigatran, rivaroxaban and apixaban showed that reduced major bleeding and intracranial bleeding rates compared to warfarin [33].

As a result, atrial fibrillation, prior or in the course of ACS, is associated with an relatively high increase in mortality and thromboembolic risk. The management of patients in acute period recieving OAC is stil debatable, especially when the patient has a coronary stent and also requires anti-platelet therapy. In the era of new oral anticoagulants and second-generation stents, it would be possible to minimize both thromboembolic events and stent thrombosis.

ACKNOWLEDGEMENTS

Declared none.

CONFLICT OF INTEREST

The authors confirm that this chapter contents have no conflict of interest.

REFERENCES

[1]　Carter CJ. The natural history and epidemiology of venous thrombosis. Prog Cardiovasc Dis 1994; 36: 423-38.

[2]　Thomas DP, Bloom AL, Forbes CD, Thomas DP, Tuddenham EGD. Pathogenesis of venous thrombosis. Haemostasis and Thrombosis, Churcill-Livingstone, New York 1994; 1335-47.

[3]　Anderson JFA, Wheeler HB, Goldberg RJ, *et al.* population-based perspective of the hospital incidence and case-fatality rates of deep vein thrombosis and pulmonary embolism: the Worcester DVT Study. Arch Intern Med 1991; 151: 933-8.

[4]   Nordstrom M, Lindblad B, Bergqvist D, Kjellstrom T. A prospective study of the incidence of deep-vein thrombosis within a defined urban population. J Intern Med 1992; 232: 155-160.

[5]   White RH. The epidemiology of venous thrombosembolism. Circulation 2003; 107: Suppl I: I-4.

[6]   Nordstrom M, Lindblad B, Bergqvist D, Kjellstrom T. A prospective study of the incidence of deep-vein thrombosis within a defined urban population. J Intern Med 1992; 232: 155-160.

[7]   Oger E. Incidence of venous thromboembolism: a community-based study in western France. Thromb Haemost 2000; 83: 657-60.

[8]   Silverstein MD, Heit JA, Mohr DN, Petterson TM, O'Fallon WM, Melton J III. Trends in the incidence of deep vein thrombosis and pulmonary embolism: a 25-year population-based study. Arch Intern Med 1998; 158: 585-93.

[9]   Heit JA, Predicting the risk of venous thromboembolism recurrence. Am J Hematol. 2012; 87 (1): 63-7.

[10]   Freiman DG. The structure of thrombi. In: Coleman RW, Hirsh J, Marder VJ, et al, (eds). Hemostasis and thrombosis: basic principles and clinical practice. 2nd Ed. Philadelphia: JB Lippincott, 1987; 1123-35

[11]   Badimon L, Badimon JJ, Fuster V. Pathogenesis of thrombosis. In: Fuster V, Verstraete M, eds. Thrombosis in cardiovascular disorders. Philadelphia: \VB Saunders, 1992; 17-39

[12]   Rosendaal FR. Venous thrombosis: a multicausal disease. Lancet 1999; 353: 1167-73.

[13]   Brouwer JLP, Veeger NJGM, Kluin-Nelemans HC. Meer J. The Pathogenesis of Venous Thromboembolism: Evidence for Multiple Interrelated Causes. Ann Intern Med. 2006; 145: 807-15.

[14]   Prandoni P, Noventa F, Ghirarduzzi A, Pengo V, Bernardi E, Pesavento R, Iotti M, Tormene D, Simioni P, Pagnan A. The risk of recurrent venous thromboembolism after discontinuing anticoagulation in patients with acute proximal deep vein thrombosis or pulmonary embolism. A prospective cohort study in 1,626 patients. Haematologica. 2007; 92: 199-205.

[15]   Hereditary and acquired antithrombin deficiency: epidemiology, pathogenesis and treatment options. Maclean PS, Tait RC. Drugs. 2007; 67(10): 1429-40.

[16]   Role of antithrombin concentrate in treatment of hereditary antithrombin deficiency. An update. Rodgers GM. Thromb Haemost. 2009; 101(5): 806-12.

[17]   Kang SS, Wong PW, Susmano A, et al. Thermolabile methylene tetrahydrofolate reductase: an inherited risk factor for coronary arter disease. Am J Hum Genet 1991; 48: 536.

[18]   Kearon C, Gent M, Hirsh J, Weitz J, Kovacs MJ, Anderson DR, Turpie AG, Green D, Ginsberg JS, Wells P, MacKinnon B, Julian JA. A comparison of three months of anticoagulation with extended anticoagulation for a first episode of idiopathic venous thromboembolism. N Engl J Med. 1999; 340: 901-7.

[19]   Zhu T, Martinez I, Emmerich J. Venous Thromboembolism Risk Factors for Recurrence. Arterioscler Thromb Vasc Biol. 2009; 29: 298-310.

[20]   Rosove MH, Brewer PM. Antiphospholipid thrombosis: clinical course after the first thrombotic event in 70 patients. Ann Intern Med. 1992; 117: 303-308.

[21]   Khamashta MA, Cuadrado MJ, Mujic F, Taub NA, Hunt BJ, Hughes GR. The management of thrombosis in the antiphospholipid-antibody syndrome. N Engl J Med. 1995; 332: 993-7.

[22]   Krnic-Barrie S, O'Connor CR, Looney SW, Pierangeli SS, Harris EN. A retrospective review of 61 patients with antiphospholipid syndrome. Analysis of factors influencing recurrent thrombosis. Arch Intern Med. 1997; 157: 2101-8.

[23]   Ageno W, Becattini C, Brighton T, Selby R, Kamphuisen PW. Cardiovascular risk factors and venous thromboembolism: a meta-analysis. Circulation. 2008; 117: 93-102.

[24]   Heit JA, Silverstein MD, Mohr DN, Petterson TM, Lohse CM, O'Fallon WM, Melton LJ, III. The epidemiology of venous thromboembolism in the community. Thromb Haemost. 2001; 86: 452-63.

[25]   Marcucci R, Liotta AA, Cellai AP, Rogolino A, Gori AM, Giusti B, Poli D, Fedi S, Abbate R, Prisco D. Increased plasma levels of lipoprotein a and the risk of idiopathic and recurrent venous thromboembolism. Am J Med. 2003; 115: 601-5.

[26]   Eichinger S, Pecheniuk NM, Hron G, Deguchi H, Schemper M, Kyrle PA, Griffin JH. High-density lipoprotein and the risk of recurrent venous thromboembolism. Circulation. 2007; 115: 1609-14.

[27]   Tsai AW, Cushman M, Rosamond WD, et al. Cardiovascular risk factors and venous thromboembolism incidence: the longitudinal investigation of thromboembolism etiology. Arch Intern Med 2002; 162: 1182.

[28]   Cushman M, Folsom AR, Wang L, *et al*. Fibrin fragment D-dimer and the risk of future venous thrombosis. Blood 2003; 101: 1243.

[29]   Poort SR, Rosendaal FR, Reitsma PH, Bertina RM, A common genetic variation in the 3' untranslated region of the prothrombin gene is associated with elevated plasma prothrombin levels and an increase in venous thrombosis. Blood 1996; 88: 3698.

[30]   Leroyer C, Mercier B, Oger E, *et al*. Prevalence of 20210 A allele of the prothrombin gene mutation in venous thromboembolism patients. Thromb Haemost 1998; 80 : 49.

[31]   De Stefano V, Martinelli I, Manucci PM, *et al*. The risk of reccurent deep venous thrombosis among heterozygous carriers of both factor V Leiden and the G20210A prothrombim mutation. N Engl J Med 1999; 341: 801.

[32]   ACTIVE Writing Group of the ACTIVE Investigators. Clopidegrol plus aspirin versus oral anticoagulation for atrial fibrillation in the atrial fibrillation clopidegrel trial with ibesartan for prevention of vascular events (ACTIVE W): a randomised controlled trial. Lancet 2006; 367: 1903-1912

[33]   Fitchett D, Verma A, Eikelboom J, *et al*. Prevention of thromboembolism in the patient with acute coronary syndrome and atrial fibrillation: the clinical dilemma of triple therapy. Curr Opin Cardiol 2014; 29: 1-9.

CHAPTER 5

Antiplatelet Resistance

Dilek Ural[*], İrem Yılmaz and Kurtuluş Karaüzüm

Kocaeli University, School of Medicine, Department of Cardiology, Umuttepe Kampüsü - 41380 Kocaeli/Türkiye

Abstract: Antiplatelet therapy is the keystone in secondary prevention of the patients with cardiovascular diseases. The efficacy of aspirin, clopidogrel and novel oral antiplatelets like prasugrel and ticagrelor in atherotrombotic events has been shown in several landmark clinical trials and meta-analyses. Nevertheless, a significant number of patients experience recurrent events despite antiplatelet therapy. Increasing evidence indicates that there is considerable variability in response to antiplatelet therapy among patients and those who have higher levels of platelet reactivity are at increased risk for recurrent ischaemic events. These findings raised the possibility that decreased response, or 'resistance' to oral antiplatelet drugs may underlie many subsequent major cardiovascular events (MACE). The main problem with 'resistance' is the lack of a clear definition. In this chapter, aspirin, clopidogrel and glycoprotein IIb/IIIa receptor inhibitor resistance in patients with acute coronary syndromes will be discussed by the concept of residual platelet activity.

Keywords: Antiplatelet, antiplatelet resistance, aspirin, clopidogrel, aspirin resistance, clopidogrel resistance, acute coronary syndrome, platelet function assays.

INTRODUCTION

Antiplatelet therapy is the keystone in secondary prevention of the patients with cardiovascular diseases. The efficacy of aspirin, clopidogrel and novel oral antiplatelets like prasugrel and ticagrelor in atherotrombotic events has been shown in several landmark clinical trials and meta-analyses [1-5]. In the latest guidelines, all of these drugs received a class I indication in acute and chronic phase (>12 months) of coronary artery syndromes [6-8]. Dual antiplatelet therapy with aspirin and a P2Y12 inhibitor (prasugrel or ticagrelor) given in the acute phase and for the following 12 months of an acute coronary syndrome is associated with improvement in long-term clinical outcomes in such patients [4, 5]. Clopidogrel is recommended for patients who cannot receive ticagrelor or prasugrel. In the chronic phase (>12 months), only aspirin is recommended for

*Corresponding author Dilek Ural: Kocaeli University, School of Medicine, Department of Cardiology Umuttepe Kampüsü - 41380 Kocaeli/Türkiye; Tel: +90 262 303 86 79; Fax: +90 262 303 87 48; E-mail: dilekural@yandex.com

Ertugrul Ercan and Gulfem Ece (Eds.)

secondary prevention unless patients are intolerant or allergic to acetylsalicylic acid. Patients who are truly intolerant to aspirin are recommended to receive clopidogrel (75 mg day) as long term secondary prevention [8]. Nevertheless, a significant number of patients experience recurrent events despite antiplatelet therapy. Increasing evidence indicates that there is considerable variability in response to antiplatelet therapy among patients and those who have higher levels of platelet reactivity are at increased risk for recurrent ischaemic events. These findings raised the possibility that decreased response, or 'resistance' to oral antiplatelet drugs may underlie many subsequent major cardiovascular events (MACE) [9].

The main problem with 'resistance' is the lack of a clear definition. Pharmacological definition of 'drug resistance' is based on the laboratory measurement of a specific target metabolite of a drug, like cAMP for clopidogrel and thromboxane for aspirin. However, clinical presentation of drug resistance is recurrence of specific events, like recurrence of ischemic events after acute coronary syndromes and in clinical practice degree of platelet function inhibition is more important than an absolute level of a metabolite. Therefore, it may be essential to replace the concept of 'resistance' with 'residual platelet reactivity' on anti-platelet treatment. In this chapter, aspirin, clopidogrel and glycoprotein IIb/IIIa receptor inhibitor resistance in patients with acute coronary syndromes will be discussed by the concept of residual platelet activity.

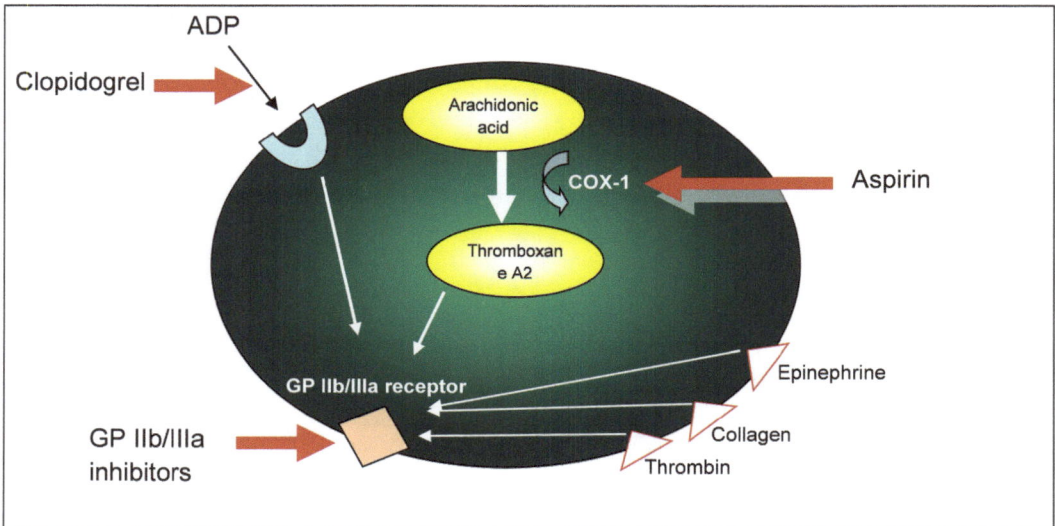

Figure 1: Sites of action of aspirin, clopidogrel and glycoprotein IIb/IIIa inhibitors.

Aspirin Resistance

Definition

Aspirin irreversibly acetylates serine residue (ser529) in COX-1 and prevents the binding of arachidonic acid to the catalytic site, which prevents the formation of thromboxane A2, a platelet activator (Fig. **1**). Aspirin may also interfere with platelet function by impairing neutrophil-mediated platelet activation [10].

Aspirin is absorbed rapidly from the gastrointestinal tract and has a half life of 20 minutes within the plasma before conversion to inactive salicylic acid. Most platelet inhibition occurs within the portal system. A single dose of aspirin can significantly inhibit 'global' platelet function within 15 minutes. The effects of aspirin on platelets continue for the lifetime of the platelet, and platelet function returns only as new platelets are formed in, and released from, the bone marrow at the rate of 10% per day [11].

From a clinical viewpoint, aspirin resistance is defined as the occurrence of thromboembolic cardiovascular events despite continued use of aspirin in therapeutic doses. However, due to the multi-factorial nature of atherothrombotic processes, the biochemical definition is more generally used. Laboratory definition of aspirin resistance is the failure of therapeutic doses of aspirin to prolong bleeding time, or a failure to reduce TXA2 production.

A formal definition of aspirin resistance has been developed by Weber *et al.*, [12] (2002) using collagen (1 mcg/ml)-induced platelet aggregation and thromboxane formation [measured as thromboxane B (2)] in citrated platelet-rich plasma. They classified aspirin resistance into three distinct pharmacokinetic and/or pharmacodynamic subtypes:

- In type 1 aspirin resistance (*pharmacokinetic*) oral treatment with aspirin is ineffective, but aspirin completely inhibits TXA2 production *in vitro*.

- In type 2 resistance (*pharmacodynamic*), aspirin fails to suppress TXA2 production both *in vitro* and *in vivo*, and

- In type 3 resistance (*pseudoresistance*), platelet activation continues despite adequate thromboxane suppression.

Although this model provides a useful tool to study the potential causes of aspirin resistance, it has no proven clinical utility.

Epidemiology

It is clear that not all patients derive the same benefit from aspirin. The prevalence of aspirin resistance shows a very wide range of variation between 0.4-57% of patients depending upon the definition and assay used, as well as the population studied [13, 14]. With optical aggregometry method aspirin resistance was found between 5.2-56.8% among the patients with coronary heart disease, whereas with a point of care system, PFA-100, which uses collagen and epinephrine as the agonists, the prevalence of aspirin resistance, is measured between 19-50% in those patients.

In a systematic review and meta-analysis, 28% of patients with cardiovascular disease were classified as aspirin resistant. Patients with aspirin resistance were at a greater risk of long term MACE than patients who are sensitive to aspirin (odds ratio 3.85, 95% confidence interval 3.08 to 4.80) [15]. Aydinalp *et al.*, [16] studied the prevalence of biochemical aspirin resistance in patients on aspirin therapy who were admitted to the emergency clinic with chest pain and found a frequency of 24%. Patients with an acute coronary syndrome had significantly more aspirin resistance than patients with rule out acute coronary syndrome or patients with stable angina pectoris (P <.001).

Etiology

The etiology of aspirin resistance is poorly understood and likely involves a combination of genetic, clinical, cellular, pharmacokinetic and pharmacodynamic factors (Table **1**).

Genetic factors - Aspirin resistance may be an inherited abnormality, especially in families with strong history of coronary heart disease. However, studies investigating genetic polymorphism as an etiology for aspirin resistance have been inconsistent. The main genetic factors for aspirin resistance include COX-1 polymorphism, over-expression of COX-2 mRNA, collagen receptor and vWF receptor polymorphisms, GP IIb/IIIa receptor polymorphism and P2Y1 single nucleotide polymorphism.

Clinical factors - Female gender, [13] advanced age, [17] metabolic syndrome, [18] diabetes mellitus (DM), [19] hypertension [20] and reduced left systolic ventricular function are all associated with a significantly higher risk of having residual platelet reactivity on treatment. Advancing age may cause a decrease in metabolism, which can predispose the elderly to underutilization of aspirin. Metabolic syndrome, DM and reduced left systolic ventricular function are conditions associated with higher platelet activity which might account for the reduced response to the drug [17, 18]. Aspirin resistance in DM is a complex interaction between a numbers of factors like inability of aspirin to inhibit COX-1 (increased protein glycation in DM reduces aspirin-mediated protein acetylation of COX-1), inflammation, prothrombotic state, increased platelet turnover and poor glycaemic control.

In patients with an acute coronary syndrome, residual platelet activity is an independent risk factor for myocardial injury and correlates with the degree of myocyte necrosis [17]. A study in STEMI patients has shown that partial inhibition of TXA2 synthesis was associated with a significant increase in myocardial injury markers, but after 48 hours post-MI, most patients achieved optimal inhibition of TXA2 by aspirin [21]. This finding suggests that aspirin resistance during an acute coronary syndrome may be a result of an inflammatory and prothrombotic condition.

The relationship between inflammation and aspirin resistance is still unclear. Not only in patients with an acute coronary event, but also patients with metabolic syndrome [22] or DM also show a relation between aspirin resistance and high inflammatory markers. Residual platelet activity related with high levels of inflammation may not be fully inhibited by standard dose of aspirin, and higher doses or other antiplatelets may be more effective in such conditions.

Cellular factors - The cellular factors like over-expression of COX-2 mRNA in vascular cells can be caused by inflammatory diseases, including atherosclerosis. COX-2 is markedly less inhibited by aspirin than COX-1. Hence, some cases of aspirin resistance may represent thromboxane generation *via* COX-2 despite successful inhibition of COX-1. Erythrocytes may also increase platelet thromboxane generation which may not be sufficiently inhibited by low to medium doses of aspirin. Increased platelet turnover in coronary heart disease could explain the ineffectiveness of low doses of ASA, since platelet TXA2 synthesis must be blocked by at least 10% for platelet inhibition to be efficient.

Pharmacokinetic and pharmacodynamic factors - Enteric coating of aspirin reduces TXB2 suppression [23]. In patients who received the enteric formulation, resistance was found in 65%, while only 25% of patients on the normal formulation demonstrated resistance. Other drugs may alter platelet function or block aspirin's acetylation of COX-1. Non steroidal antiinflammatory drugs (NSAIDs) reversibly inhibit COX-1 by 70-90% at conventional doses. Several studies have assessed the effect of the interaction between ibuprofen and aspirin;

ibuprofen given 2 hours prior to aspirin markedly reduces inhibition of TXB2 release in comparison to aspirin being given 2 hours before ibuprofen (p<0.001) [3]. Studies about the effect of statins on aspirin resistance results with conflicting findings. While some studies proposed statin use as an independent risk factor for aspirin resistance, [24] other have suggested that lowering of lipid levels with statins results in low frequency of aspirin resistance.

Table 1: Factors contributing aspirin resistance

Clinical factors	Cellular factors	Genetic factors
• Non-compliance • Non-absorption • Old age • Female gender • Smoking • Acute coronary syndrome • Congestive heart failure • Metabolic syndrome • Obesity • Diabetes • Interaction with other drugs • Catecholamine surge	• Insufficient suppression of COX-1 • Over expression of COX-2 mRNA • Erythrocyte induced platelet activation • Increased norepinephrine • Generation of 8-iso-PGF 2α	• COX-1 polymorphism • GP IIb/IIIa receptor polymorphism • Collagen receptor polymorphisms • vWF receptor polymorphisms

Detecting Aspirin Resistance

Assessing aspirin resistance is a debated subject; because there is considerable heterogeneity among the many *in vitro* assays available. Lordkipanidzé *et al.*, [25] compared the results obtained from six major platelet function tests in the assessment of the prevalence of aspirin resistance in 201 patients with stable coronary artery disease receiving daily aspirin therapy (> or =80 mg). The prevalence of aspirin resistance varied according to the assay used from 6.7% for VerifyNow Aspirin to 59.5% for PFA-100. The authors concluded that platelet function tests are not equally effective in measuring aspirin's antiplatelet effect and correlate poorly amongst themselves. The reason for the poor correlation between the various *in vitro* assays is the heterogeneity of their designs; they utilize the tendency of platelets to change shape, aggregate, release metabolic products, or mobilize cell-surface receptors upon activation [26].

The only *in vivo* measure of platelet function is bleeding time but it is also poorly reproducible and has several confounding variables such as platelet count and degree of injury to both vessels and tissues [27].

Characteristics, advantages and disadvantages of the most frequently used *in vitro* platelet function assays are summarized below (Table **2**).

Table 2: *In vitro* aspirin resistance/platelet function assays

Assay	Sample type	Advantages	Disadvantages
Light transmittance aggregometry (LTA)	Platelet rich plasma Whole blood	Accepted as the gold standard Measures directly platelet aggregation Shows good correlation with clinical events	Labour intensive and expensive Difficult to standardize Poorly reproducible
VerifyNow®	Whole blood	Point of care test Best reproducibility Shows good correlation with clinical events	Expensive
Platelet function analyzer (PFA)-100	Whole blood	Point of care test Shows good correlation with clinical events	Poorly reproducible Not specific for aspirin resistance No defined cut-off closure time for aspirin resistance Dependent upon vWF and haematocrit
Urinary/serum thromboxane B2	Urine or serum	Depends on COX inhibition Shows good correlation with clinical events	Poorly reproducible Not specific for COX-1 inhibition Not specific for aspirin resistance

Light Transmission Aggregometry (LTA): LTA allows more precise quantification of platelet aggregation than the other assays and is considered as the gold standard. It measures the increase in light transmission after the aggregation of platelets suspended in plasma in response to various agonists such as arachidonic acid, collagen, epinephrine or adenosine diphosphate (ADP). This assay commonly isolates platelets from other constituents (leukocytes and erythrocytes) of platelet aggregation in plasma, although whole-blood aggregometry may also be used. For the assessment of aspirin resistance, platelet aggregation is measured in response to arachidonic acid. Although LTA is advantageous as a direct method for platelet aggregation assessment, using only arachidonic acid may also be a disadvantage as other agonists, like ADP and epinephrine are not considered.

LTA is also operator and interpreter dependent and it is difficult to standardize measures across different laboratories due to variations in sampling techniques, centrifugation and preparation of platelet rich plasma.

Whole blood aggregometry (WBA) is a similar method to LTA. Changes in electrical impedance during platelet aggregation in whole blood are measured. The main advantage over LTA is less sample preparation. However, correlation between WBA and LTA is poor [26].

The VerifyNow® system (Accumetrics, USA) is a point of care system for the rapid detection of platelet aggregation. Three different VerifyNow systems are available for the assessment of aspirin, P2Y12 antagonists, and GPIIb/IIIa antagonists resistance. The VerifyNow aspirin system uses turbidimetric optical detection of platelet aggregation to fibrinogen and arachidonic acid in whole blood. Changes in light transmittance during platelet aggregation are measured and converted into Aspirin Reaction Units (ARU) with a pre-defined value for aspirin resistance of greater than 550 ARU [26]. Its sensitivity, specificity, positive and negative productivity compared to LTA as the gold standard is 38%, 95%, 23% and 97% respectively [26].

The Platelet Function Analyzer (PFA)-100 system - The PFA-100 (Sysmex) assesses platelet aggregation using disposable cartridges that mimics thrombus formation in a small caliber injured blood vessel. Whole blood is passed through a small orifice made of collagen and epinephrine or collagen and ADP-coated membrane under high shear stress. The time necessary to close a microscopic aperture [closure time (CT)] in a membrane coated with collagen and epinephrine (CEPI) or ADP (CADP) is measured, and is used to define the presence of aspirin resistance [28]. The CEPI cartridges are considered to be COX-dependent and are thought to detect qualitative changes in platelet function including aspirin-induced dysfunction. Whereas, the CADP cartridges are COX-independent, therefore relatively ineffective at detecting aspirin inhibitory effects and are generally used as a test of thienopyridine response. There is no definite cut-off value to define aspirin resistance and CT <171-200 s are accepted as aspirin resistance in different studies [29].

Although the PFA-100 is one of the most widely used tests of aspirin response, there are many concerns about it. PFA-100 was originally developed as a measure of platelet function in hematological disease (*e.g.,* von Willebrand Disease) and is not specific for COX-1 inhibition. Results from the PFA-100 may be confused by other hematological variables which are not involved in the response of aspirin such as vWF, haematocrit and platelet count. PFA-100 also poorly correlates with other measures of platelet function and reports prevalence of aspirin resistance higher than the other assays. Its sensitivity, specificity, positive and negative predictivity compared to LTA as the gold standard is 75%, 40%, 5% and 97% respectively [26].

Urine 11-dehydrothromboxane B2 (Ur 11dhTXB2) - Arachidonic acid is converted to prostaglandins including thromboxane A2 by cyclooxygenase. Inhibition of the activation of COX-1 by aspirin results with the decreased production of thromboxane A2 (TXA2). TXB2 is a stable metabolite of TXA2 and therefore could be regarded as a direct measure of COX-1 inhibition by aspirin. Ur 11dhTXB2 can easily be measured from the urine by ELISA [30].

Elevated Ur 11dhTXB2 is associated with a greater cardiovascular risk factor profile which is consistent with previous findings that the severity of atherosclerotic disease may modify thromboxane generation independent of aspirin *via* increased COX-2 expression [31]. Lack of suppression of Ur11 dhTXB2 may not always represent aspirin resistance; instead it may be a marker of aspirin insensitive thromboxane generation *via* other mechanisms despite adequate inhibition of platelet COX-1 activity by aspirin. However, Ur 11dhTXB2 levels can be variable because they are dependent on the rate and volume of urine collected.

Other methods - Plateletworks$^{®}$ is a relatively novel point of care test for aspirin response. It assesses whole blood platelet aggregation *via* comparison of a baseline platelet count and platelet count following addition of arachidonic acid as an agonist, and values are expressed either as % platelet inhibition or % platelet aggregation. Platelet activation can also be determined by flow cytometry [32]. The two most commonly used flow cytometric markers of platelet activation are those directed against the glycoprotein GPIIb-IIIa (The PAC1 monoclonal antibody) and the adhesion protein P-selectin. Flow cytometry has the advantage of directly measuring platelet activation, but it is expensive and is not available in many laboratories. Measurement of soluble P-selectin or serum 11-dehydrothromboxane B2 may also reflect the level of platelet activation.

The position paper from the Working Group on antiplatelet drugs resistance of the Polish Cardiac Society proposed the reference test to evaluate *functional* resistance to aspirin as platelet aggregation induced by arachidonic acid with the use of optical transmittance aggregometry and the most reliable *biochemical* test as measurement of serum levels of TXB2 [33].

Management

As mentioned above, clinical definition of platelet resistance is the lack of the desired pharmacologic effect of an antiplatelet medication. However, the occurrence of an ischaemic clinical event while taking an antiplatelet therapy does not necessarily indicate that resistance is present. Besides, routine evaluation of resistance is still not recommended. Nevertheless, aspirin resistance is an issue with potentially important public health implications because of aspirins' established role in secondary prevention. Patients must be evaluated in terms of compliance and interacting medications regularly. Some patients with persistent platelet reactivity despite treatment with aspirin may simply be non-compliant to their medications. In addition, stopping interacting medications, such as NSAIDs, may be of benefit. It is uncertain that increasing the dose of aspirin based on laboratory evidence of aspirin resistance will be clinically beneficial. Neubauer *et al.*, [34] evaluated the effect of increasing aspirin dose in a post-PCI group in whom resistance was detected using whole blood aggregometry. In a prespecified tailored therapy algorithm, they increased aspirin dose in low responders from 100 mg to 300 mg in the first step or to 500 mg ASA when the first modification did not take effect sufficiently. After dose adjustment, all initial low responders had an adequate antiplatelet response. However, the long-term follow-up results of treating laboratory resistance were not evaluated. In a sub-study of the CHARISMA trial [35], it has been demonstrated that there is no clear benefit of in giving aspirin in doses greater than 100 mg/day and there is a non-significant trend to increased harm from both cardiovascular events and bleeding at higher doses particularly in diabetic patients. The mechanisms behind this are unclear, but may reflect a reduction in prostacyclin production, a powerful COX-dependent vasodilator, as a result of higher aspirin doses or poor compliance with aspirin therapy due to increased side-effects at higher doses.

Adding a different antiplatelet drug such as clopidogrel or dipyridamole has been suggested as a method to treat aspirin resistant patients. Still, no clinical trial exists to show the effectiveness of this approach, and although not specifically performed in aspirin resistant patients, trials with prolonged dual antiplatelet therapy after coronary stenting did not show any additional benefit beyond 1 year [36].

Larger clinical trials with long-term follow up are needed to confirm if it is beneficial and safe to add a different antiplatelet drug. For now, additional antiplatelet drugs should only be prescribed in patients who experience recurrent vascular events despite taking aspirin, where there is good evidence that the patient will benefit (post acute coronary syndrome, MI or stroke).

Future research should focus on how aspirin resistance should be detected, predicted and managed. Predicting low aspirin response in patients, who need antiplatelet therapy as secondary prevention, may have the great clinical utility in reducing cardiovascular mortality and morbidity.

Clopidogrel Resistance

Definition

Clopidogrel is a second-generation thienopyridine that binds to the platelet surface $P2Y_{12}$ ADP receptor irreversibly and inhibits ADP-induced platelet activation (Fig. **1**). It is an inactive prodrug that needs conversion to an active metabolite by the cytochrome P450 3A4 enzyme system in the liver. Although the latest acute coronary syndrome guidelines recommend novel ADP receptors blockers, prasugrel and ticagrelor, more preferably than clopidogrel because of their more rapid onset of action, greater potency and proved superiority in large outcome trials, clopidogrel is still widely used because of its known clinical profile and lower cost.

There is variability between patients with regard to clopidogrel-induced inhibition of platelet function. Clopidogrel resistance is defined as a relative lack of clopidogrel induced $P2Y_{12}$ inhibition in platelet function assays. In clinical setting, clopidogrel resistance is characterized by the occurrence of thrombotic events despite clopidogrel therapy. Variable responsiveness to clopidogrel has required the development of novel $P2Y_{12}$ inhibitors with superior pharmacodynamic profiles as mentioned above [37].

Epidemiology and Etiology

The prevalence of clopidogrel resistance varies from 5-44% of patients with coronary artery disease depending upon the clinical scenario, test assay and clopidogrel dose [38].

Clopidogrel is a prodrug that is metabolized by cytochrome P450 into an active metabolite. Only 15% of the dose of clopidogrel absorbed is metabolized in the active drug, especially by cytochrome P3A4 (CYP3A4) [39]. Possible causes of decreased responsiveness to the clopidogrel include genetic polymorphisms of the platelet $P2Y_{12}$ ADP receptor, defects in signaling pathways downstream from the receptor, heightened platelet reactivity before drug administration, body mass index or comorbidities (*e.g.*, insulin resistance, heart failure) (Table **2** and Fig. **2**) [40].

Genetic factors - Because the response to clopidogrel shows wide variation among individuals, many studies have been conducted to investigate possible genetic factors that may predispose to these differences (Table **3**). It appears that the main cause of variation originates from clopidogrel metabolism and main factors are polymorphisms in hepatic cytochrome P450 isozymes (*e.g.*, CYP3A4, CYP3A5, and CYP2C19) and in the $P2Y_{12}$ receptor itself.

Table 2: Factors contributing clopidogrel resistance

Genetic factors	Cellular factors	Clinical factors
• Polymorphisms of glycoprotein Ia and IIIa genes • Polymorphisms of the P-450 CYP3A gene • Polymorphisms of the $P2Y_{12}$ gene	• Accelerated platelet turnover and increased platelet production by the bone marrow • Increased baseline platelet reactivity • Up-regulation of $P2Y_{12}$ and other ($P2Y_1$, collagen, epinephrine, thromboxane A_2, thrombin) platelet pathways • Reduced cytochrome P-450 CYP3A4 metabolic activity	• Failure to prescribe • Poor compliance • Inadequate dose (perhaps in ACS or stenting) • Poor absorption • Increased metabolism • Drug interactions involving CYP3A4 • Diabetes mellitus • insulin resistance • Obesity • Heart failure

In terms of polymorphisms in CYP2C19, loss-of-function polymorphisms were first shown to significantly reduce the response to clopidogrel in platelets from healthy subjects, as demonstrated by increased platelet aggregation measured using light transmission aggregometry [41]. The prevalence of poor metabolizers or intermediate metabolizers of clopidogrel are higher in Asian (18-23%) than in Caucasian (approximately 3%) populations, and this may be related to the common gene variants of CYP2C19 in these populations [42].

Cellular factors - A high platelet turnover rate leads to an increase in the number of immature reticulated platelets that could confer residual platelet reactivity, despite of clopidogrel use. In times of stress, the bone marrow has accelerated platelet production. These platelets carry $P2Y_{12}$ receptors that are unexposed to clopidogrel, which leads to an indirect clopidogrel resistance.

Clinical factors - Among the many clinical factors responsible for clopidogrel resistance, increased metabolism originating from drug-drug interaction is the most frequently studied factor. Theoretically, concurrent medication use may interfere with the ability of clopidogrel to decrease platelet reactivity. High doses of calcium channel blockers and angiotensin converting enzyme inhibitors possibly contribute to a depleted response to clopidogrel [43]. Atorvastatin is the most frequently studied lipophilic statin in clopidogrel trials because it has a high affinity for CYP3A4. Schmidt *et al.,* [44] examined whether CYP3A4-metabolizing statin use modified the association between clopidogrel use and major adverse cardiovascular events after coronary stenting. In a population-based cohort study in Western Denmark using medical databases, they have not observed any interaction between statin use and clopidogrel and increased rate of events.

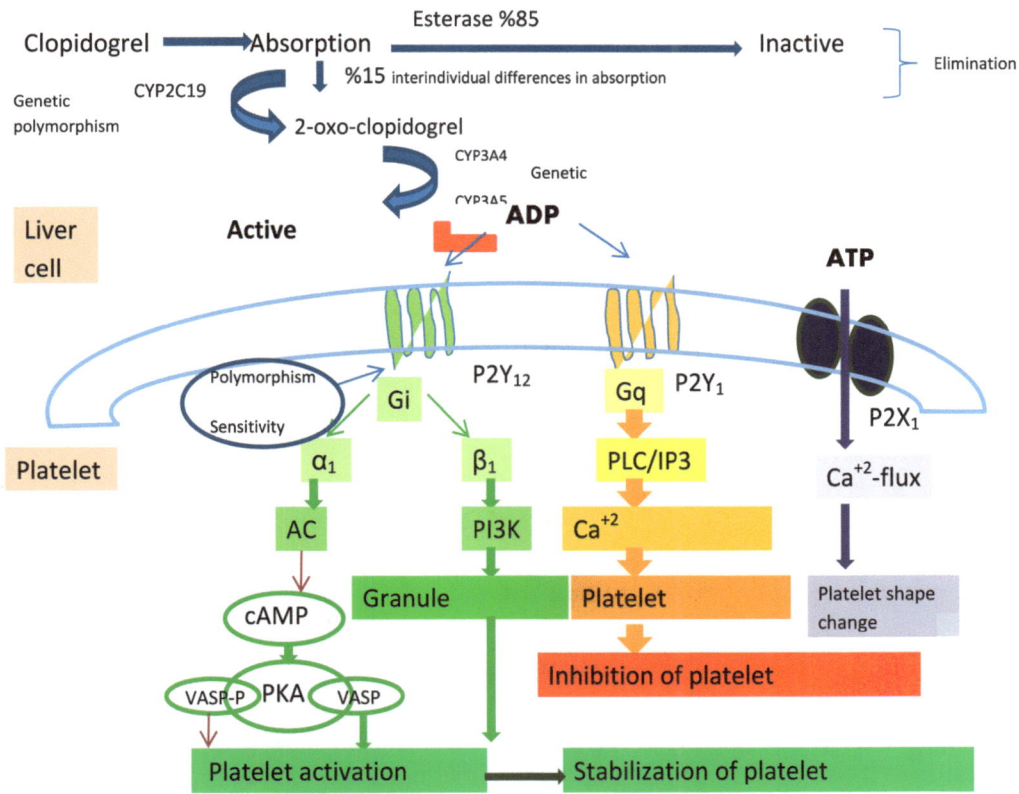

Figure 2: Pathways and possible mechanisms involved in response to clopidogrel. AC, adenylate cyclase; ADP, adenosine diphosphate; AMP, adenosine monophosphates; ATP, adenosine triphosphate; cAMP, cyclic adenosine monophosphate; CYP, cytochrome P450; Gi, inhibitory G protein; Gq, stimulatory G protein; IP3, inositol triphosphate; PDE, phosphodiesterase; PKA, protein kinase A; VASP, vasodilator-stimulated phosphoprotein; PI3K, phosphatidyl inositol 3-kinase; PLC, phospholipase C.

CYP2C9, CYP2C19 and CYP1A2 are involved in the transformation of clopidogrel to the active drug. Proton pump inhibitors that inhibit CYP2C19, particularly omeprazole, decrease clopidogrel-induced platelet inhibition *ex vivo*, but there is currently no conclusive clinical evidence that co-administration of clopidogrel and proton pump inhibitors increases the risk of ischaemic events [45]. One randomized trial (prematurely interrupted for lack of funding) tested routine omeprazole combined with clopidogrel *vs.* clopidogrel alone in patients with an indication for dual antiplatelet therapy (DAPT) for 12 months, including post-PCI patients, ACS, or other indications. No increase in ischaemic event rates but a reduced rate of upper gastrointestinal bleeding was observed with omeprazole. Interindividual variability in baseline activity of the hepatic cytochrome P-450 CYP3A4 system may also influence clopidogrel metabolism [46]. Lau *et al.*, [47] showed that platelet inhibition was enhanced when rifampin, a CYP3A4 inducer, was administered with clopidogrel.

The absorption of clopidogrel is regulated by multidrug-resistance protein 1 (MDR1) in the intestinal epithelium. Tauber and colleagues [48] demonstrated that the intestinal absorption is the main factor determining the production of active metabolites of clopidogrel. Also ISAR-CHOICE study compared the effects of clopidogrel on the inhibition of platelet function at higher loading doses (300, 600 and 900 mg) and demonstrated that there are no advantages in doses higher than 600 mg, as this does not result in a corresponding higher level of active metabolite in plasma [49]. This finding suggests that intestinal absorption is reduced for doses higher than 600 mg.

Acute coronary syndrome is characterized by an enhanced platelet reactivity caused by a higher platelet turn-over, documented by the presence of reticulated platelets which are another determinant of the entity of platelet inhibition [50]. Matezky *et al.*, [51] presented the first study suggesting the impact of clopidogrel-induced antiplatelet effects on post-stent ischaemic events in patients of ST elevation MI following PCI. In this study, 60 patients were randomized to 4 groups according to the percentage reduction of ADP-induced platelet aggregation. In the first quartile, 40% of patients sustained a recurrent cardiovascular event (STEMI, acute coronary syndrome, subacute stent thrombosis, and acute arterial occlusion) during 6-month follow-up, only 1 patient (6.7%) in the second quartile and none of the third and fourth quartiles experienced a cardiovascular event (p = 0.007). A recent study evaluated responsiveness to clopidogrel in 804 consecutive patients receiving sirolimus or paclitaxel -eluting stents. All patients received aspirin (325 mg) and a loading dose of 600 mg of clopidogrel followed by a maintenance dose of 75 mg daily; 13% of patients were not responsive to clopidogrel [52]. At 6 months, the incidence of stent thrombosis was 8.6% in nonresponders and 2.3% in responders ($p < 0.001$). By multivariate analysis, nonresponsiveness to clopidogrel was a strong independent predictor of stent thrombosis (hazard ratio 3.08, 95% confidence interval 1.32 to 7.16, $p = 0.009$). Patients with unstable angina undergoing PCI demonstrate lower inhibition of platelet aggregation following clopidogrel loading compared to patients with stable angina [53]. Another important study to document this was the CREST (Clopidogrel Effect on Platelet Reactivity in Patients with Stent Thrombosis) study. This study showed that high post-treatment platelet reactivity and incomplete $P2Y_{12}$ were risk factors for subacute stent thrombosis. These findings suggest that patients presenting with acute coronary syndromes are a subgroup of patients with an increased likelihood of clopidogrel resistance.

Diabetes, obesity and reduced systolic ventricular function are associated with a significantly higher prevalence of residual platelet reactivity on therapy [17]. Diabetes and heart failure are also known to be associated with higher platelet reactivity. Finally, inflammation, measured by white cells number, erythrocyte sedimentation rate and the balance between pro and anti-inflammatory cytokines in diabetes, acute coronary syndromes and heart failure has been demonstrated to be a predictor of on-therapy platelet reactivity [17, 48].

Detection and Measuring Clopidogrel Resistance

A standardized laboratory method that simulates the *in vivo* platelet response to antiplatelet therapy is still lacking. Platelet function, and hence clopidogrel activity, can be measured *in vitro* using a number of different approaches. The most commonly used approaches include ADP-induced platelet aggregation, VASP phosphorylation/flow cytometry, thromboelastography, the platelet drop-count method, and light transmission elastography.

Light transmission aggregometry - As stated in aspirin resistance, the historical gold standard method is light transmission aggregometry (turbidometric) (LTA). In this method, blood samples that readily aggregate (*e.g.,* in the absence of a platelet inhibitor or those containing platelets that are nonresponsive to clopidogrel) show high light transmittance because the aggregates fall out solution and impaired responses to platelet inhibitors are measured as a decrease in light transmission relative platelet-poor plasma samples. Normal values for platelet reactivity are <42.9% to 5 μmol/L ADP and <64.5% to 20 μmol/L ADP. Cut-off value to define high platelet reactivity is >46% to 5 µmol/L ADP. Although this approach is considered the 'gold standard' for measuring platelet reactivity, it is not specific for the $P2Y_{12}$ pathway.

The VerifyNow^{TM} assay (Accumetrics, San Diego, CA, USA) - VerifyNow system is based on light transmission aggregometry and, in contrast to LTA, is specific for the $P2Y_{12}$ pathway. Compared with standard LTA, the VerifyNow assay measures an increase in light transmission to indicate increased aggregation, as the coated beads that bind to the aggregates fall out of solution. The cut-off $P2Y_{12}$ reaction units (PRU) to detect resistance is >235. The VerifyNow assay has been used in several studies to investigate the prevalence of aspirin and clopidogrel resistance [54]. Furthermore, it seems that this system is more reliable than other methods, like the platelet drop count method or thromboelastography [55].

It was initially considered that ADP-induced platelet aggregation could be used as a marker for clopidogrel activity. However, clopidogrel specifically inhibits the $P2Y_{12}$ receptor rather than the P2Y1 receptor, which is responsible for the initial wave of ADP-induced platelet aggregation. Furthermore, because the extent of residual P2Y1-dependent platelet aggregation varies considerably, ADP-induced aggregation may not be the most appropriate method to measure the response to clopidogrel. Therefore, other approaches have been evaluated. In thromboelastography, a small blood sample is placed in a cuvette and aggregation is induced by gentle rotation or injection of ADP [56]. The platelet-fibrin clot strength of the clot is weak, whereas in platelets exhibiting resistance to clopidogrel, the strength of the clots will be greater.

The platelet count drop method is widely available in the laboratories. However, it is not clear whether this approach provides significant clinical information, and it seems to be less reliable than LTA [57].

Vasodilator stimulated phosphoprotein (VASP) phosphorylation - This method specifically focuses on the $P2Y_{12}$ pathway, which leads to the phosphorylation of VASP and assesses biochemical effect of clopidogrel. The phosphorylation state of VASP is evaluable by flow $P2Y_{12}$ receptor reactivity in patients on clopidogrel. The cut-off value for resistance is variable among the studies, but a 'platelet reactivity index (PRI)' >50% is generally considered as a limit related to increased cardiovascular events. However, flow cytometers may not be readily available, particularly in a point-of-care setting and are expensive. Accordingly, a number of point-of-care assays have been developed to provide rapid assessment of the potential for clopidogrel resistance in a clinical setting.

Breet *et al.*, [58] compared the abilities of several widely used techniques for measuring on-treatment platelet reactivity (LTA, VerifyNow P2Y12, PlateletWorks, IMPACT-R, and the PFA-100 platelet function analysis system) to predict the clinical outcomes of 1069 patients taking clopidogrel and undergoing elective coronary stent implantation. The primary endpoint, a composite of all-cause death, nonfatal acute MI, stent thrombosis and ischaemic stroke at 1 year, occurred more frequently in patients with high on-treatment platelet activity, when assessed by LTA, VerifyNow, PlateletWorks and Innovance PFA P2Y which were able to discriminate between patients with or without a primary event. The other techniques were not able to discriminate between these two groups of patients. Meanwhile, the authors reported that the predictive accuracy of these four tests was only modest. None of the tests provided accurate prognostic information to identify patients at higher risk of bleeding following stent implantation.

Management

The response to clopidogrel appears to be time dependent and decreases with prolonged use [59]. Subsequent investigations have clearly demonstrated that clopidogrel nonresponsiveness is dependent on dose [60]. Therefore two main methods to overcome clopidogrel resistance are clopidogrel dose increase and change of clopidogrel with other antiplatelets with more rapid onset of action.

Clopidogrel Dose Increase

The first option in patients with clopidogrel resistance may be to increase the dose of clopidogrel. In clinical use, clopidogrel is commonly administered at a loading dose of 600 mg. Several studies have documented importance of adequate dose of loading in acute coronary settings and prior to PCI [61-64].

Current maintenance dose of clopidogrel is 75 mg/day. This dose was chosen because the degree of platelet inhibition is similar to that achieved by ticlopidine 25 mg BID. Cuisset *et al.*, [65] evaluated the benefit of tailored therapy with a higher maintenance dose according to CYP2C19 genotypes in patients identified as nonresponders who underwent PCI for non-ST-segment elevation acute coronary syndromes. All clopidogrel nonresponders received high 150-mg clopidogrel maintenance doses at discharge to overcome initial low response. After 1 month, high maintenance doses overcame clopidogrel low response in only 44% of the whole population and significantly less frequently in *2 carriers than in noncarriers (28% *vs.* 50%, p = 0.01). The authors concluded that higher clopidogrel maintenance doses could overcome clopidogrel low response in less than half percent of low responders and CYP2C19*2 carrier patients might require alternative strategies with new P2Y$_{12}$ blockers. Han *et al.*, [66] evaluated the short-term efficacy and safety of a 150 mg maintenance dose of clopidogrel following a 600 mg loading dose in patients with an acute coronary syndrome undergoing drug eluting stent implantation. At a follow-up period of 30 days, 4 (1.0%) patients in the 150 mg group and 9 (2.2%) patients in the 75 mg group (P >0.05) reached the primary end points defined as the composite of cardiac death, non-fatal myocardial infarction (MI) and urgent target vessel revascularization. There was no significant difference in the incidence of MI (0.5% *vs.* 1.2%, P > 0.05) and cardiac death (0.2% *vs.* 0.2%, P > 0.05) between the two groups. There were no significant differences between both groups regarding the risk of major or minor bleedings. Similarly Aradi *et al.*, [67] also showed that administration of 150 mg clopidogrel significantly reduced platelet aggregation in clopidogrel-naive stable angina patients with high platelet reactivity (AGGmax ≥34%) before and after percutaneous coronary intervention. The higher maintenance dose of clopidogrel was associated with a significant reduction in cardiovascular death and myocardial infarction (0% *vs.* 11·4%, P = 0·04) during 1 year.

The OPTIMUS (Optimizing anti-Platelet Therapy In diabetes MellitUS) study [68] selectively studied diabetes mellitus patients with high post-treatment platelet reactivity while in their chronic phase of treatment. In these patients, although a 150 mg clopidogrel maintenance dose resulted in marked platelet inhibition of numerous platelet function measures compared with a 75 mg dose, a considerable number of patients still remained above the therapeutic threshold of post-treatment platelet reactivity used in this study, suggesting the need for more potent P2Y12 inhibitors or alternative antithrombotic regimens in these high-risk patients.

Taken together, the findings of these studies indicate the potential for using higher maintenance doses of clopidogrel. However, the efficacy of increasing the clopidogrel dose is of limited benefit, and many patients may need another antiplatelet agent to overcome residual platelet activity. Pharmacogenetic analysis may be useful for the decision to use high-dose clopidogrel or switching to another antiplatelet agent. In the RESET-GENE trial [69] high on-treatment platelet reactivity could successfully be abolished by high-dose clopidogrel in CYP2C19*2 noncarriers but not in CYP2C19*2 carriers. Efficacy of prasugrel was not effected by genotype in that study.

Alternative Drugs

Prasugrel is a novel antiplatelet agent that targets the ADP receptor in platelets. The efficacy of prasugrel has been compared with that of clopidogrel in several studies. In the TRITON-TIMI-38 study, [5] 13.608 patients with moderate-to-high risk ACS scheduled to undergo PCI were randomized to either prasugrel (60-mg loading dose; 10-mg daily maintenance dose) or clopidogrel (300-mg loading dose; 75-mg daily maintenance dose for 6-15 months). The primary end point (death from cardiovascular causes or nonfatal MI or stroke) occurred in significantly fewer patients treated with prasugrel than patients treated with clopidogrel (9.9% *vs*. 12.1%, respectively; HR = 0,81; 95% CI= 0.73-0.90; *P* < 0.001). In the PRINCIPLE-TIMI 44 study, [70] 201 subjects were treated with either prasugrel (60-mg loading dose followed by 10 mg/day) or high-dose clopidogrel (600-mg loading dose followed by 150 mg/day) for inhibition of platelet aggregation and aggregation-thrombolysis in MI. The primary end point in this study was the inhibition of platelet aggregation (in response to 20 μmol/L ADP) at the end of the loading-dose phase, and observed significantly higher with prasugrel than with clopidogrel (61.3% *vs*. 46.1%; *P* < 0.001). A subsequent analysis of the study showed that the intrinsic platelet response to adenosine diphosphate (ADP) before thienopyridine exposure contributed to residual platelet reactivity to ADP despite high level $P2Y_{12}$ blockade by prasugrel or high-dose clopidogrel. This finding suggested that a small number of patients may still show antiplatelet resistance despite prasugrel therapy, which was approved by ACAPULCO study, [71] that showed a 0-6% residual platelet activity in ACS patients treated with prasugrel 10 mg compared to 4-34% residual activity in those treated with clopidogrel using 900 mg loading dose continued with 150 mg maintenance dose.

Efficacy of prasugrel was also superior to high-dose clopidogrel in patients undergoing PCI or having stable coronary artery disease and diabetes [72, 73].

Ticagrelor is another novel antiplatelet agent that binds to $P2Y_{12}$ to antagonize the ADP receptor on platelets, and inhibits platelet aggregation. However, unlike clopidogrel, ticagrelor binds to $P2Y_{12}$ reversibly and does not displace ADP from the receptor, targeting 2-MeS-ADP-induced signaling. In addition, ticagrelor does not require hepatic enzymatic activation, and thus may provide more consistent platelet inhibition with reduced risk for drug interactions. Ticagrelor action is unlikely to be affected by CYP polymorphisms. Ticagrelor efficacy in ACS was studied in the PLATelet inhibition and patient Outcomes (PLATO) trial [4]. In this study 18,624 patients admitted with an ACS, with or without ST-segment elevation, were randomized to receive either ticagrelor (180-mg loading dose plus 90 mg twice daily thereafter) or clopidogrel (300-600-mg loading dose plus 75 mg daily thereafter). At 12 months, the primary endpoint (a composite of death from vascular causes, MI or stroke) occurred in 9.8% of patients treated with ticagrelor *vs.* 11.8% of those treated with clopidogrel (HR = 0.84; 95% CI = 0.77-0.92; $P < 0.001$). However, ticagrelor was associated with increased rates of ventricular pauses and mild-to-moderate dyspnea, although the underlying cause could not been established. Efficacy of ticagrelor was indirectly compared with high-dose clopidogrel and prasugrel in a meta-analysis [74]. No difference was found between the three treatment options in terms of all cause mortality, cardiovascular mortality, MI and stroke. Stent thrombosis was found to be lower with prasugrel compared to high-dose clopidogrel and ticagrelor (OR 0.68 and 0.63, respectively), but major or minor bleeding occurred more frequently with prasugrel than with ticagrelor (OR 1.37; 95% CI 1.11-1.68). However, ticagrelor was associated with less major or minor bleeding compared to high-dose clopidogrel (OR 0.81, 95% CI 0.69-0.96).

Cilostazol inhibits platelet aggregation by antagonizing the activity of phosphodiesterase III and thereby suppresses cAMP degradation in platelets. Cilostazol has been suggested to offer an alternative approach for patients with clopidogrel resistance. Accordingly, the efficacy and safety of cilostazol in combination with clopidogrel and aspirin *versus* clopidogrel plus aspirin has been investigated in several ACS studies [75, 76]. Collectively, adjunctive cilostazol to dual antiplatelet therapy ('triple antiplatelet therapy') has a potential to reduce ischemic event occurrence compared with standard dual antiplatelet therapy. Thus in patients with low response to clopidogrel therapy, adding cilostazol may be more effective than high maintenance doses of clopidogrel [77, 78]. However, current studies include relatively small numbers of patients and are of short durations, limiting a detailed analyses of endpoints such death or incidence of major cardiovascular events. Thus, further studies are needed to confirm these findings.

Glycoprotein IIb/IIIa Resistance

The GpIIb/IIIa antagonists (abciximab, eptifibatide and tirofiban) inhibit fibrinogen binding to platelet surface GpIIb/IIIa (integrin $\alpha IIb\beta 3$), the final common pathway of platelet aggregation. There is a substantial patient-to-patient variability in the degree of inhibition of platelet function by GpIIb/IIIa antagonists and an *in vitro* test of abciximab resistance (VerifyNow®) can predict MACE [79]. However, unlike for aspirin resistance and clopidogrel resistance, no published studies address the clinical effectiveness of alternating therapy based on GpIIb/IIIa antagonist resistance.

Although antiplatelet resistance is an important contributor to recurrent events in patients with known cardiovascular disease, current consensus on the routine evaluation and management of this condition in not clearly established. Antiplatelet resistance will be one of the most important applications of pharmacogenetics to guide choosing agents with the greatest potential of efficacy and smallest risk of adverse drug reactions.

ACKNOWLEDGEMENTS

Declared none.

CONFLICT OF INTEREST

The authors confirm that this chapter contents have no conflict of interest.

REFERENCES

[1]   Baigent C, Blackwell L, Collins R, *et al.* Aspirin in the primary and secondary prevention of vascular disease: collaborative meta-analysis of individual participant data from randomised trials. Lancet 2009; 373: 1849-1860.
[2]   Investigators TCT. Effects of clopidogrel in addition to aspirin in patients with acute coronary syndromes without ST-segment elevation. N Engl J Med 2001; 345: 494-502.
[3]   Chen ZM, Jiang LX, Chen YP, Xie JX, Pan HC, Peto R, Collins R, Liu LS. Addition of clopidogrel to aspirin in 45,852 patients with acute myocardial infarction: randomised placebo-controlled trial. Lancet 2005; 366: 1607-1621.
[4]   Wallentin L, Becker RC, Budaj A, *et al.* Ticagrelor *versus* clopidogrel in patients with acute coronary syndromes. N Engl J Med 2009; 361: 1045-1057.
[5]   Wiviott SD, Braunwald E, McCabe CH, Montalescot G, Ruzyllo W, Gottlieb S, Neumann FJ, *et al*; TRITON-TIMI 38 Investigators. Prasugrel *versus* clopidogrel in patients with acute coronary syndromes. N Engl J Med 2007; 357: 2001-15.
[6]   Perk J, De Backer G, Gohlke H, Graham I, Reiner Z, Verschuren M, *et al.* European Guidelines on cardiovascular disease prevention in clinical practice (version 2012). Eur Heart J 2012; 33: 1635-701.
[7]   Hamm CW, Bassand JP, Agewall S, Bax J, Boersma E, Bueno H, Caso P, *et al.* ESC Guidelines for the management of acute coronary syndromes in patients presenting without persistent ST-segment elevation: The Task Force for the management of acute coronary syndromes (ACS) in patients presenting without persistent ST-segment elevation of the European Society of Cardiology (ESC). Eur Heart J 2011; 32: 2999-3054.
[8]   Authors/Task Force Members, Steg PG, James SK, Atar D, Badano LP, Lundqvist CB, Borger MA, *et al.* ESC Guidelines for the management of acute myocardial infarction in patients presenting with ST-segment elevation: The Task Force on the management of ST-segment elevation acute myocardial infarction of the European Society of Cardiology (ESC). Eur Heart J 2012; 33: 2569-619.
[9]   Cuisset T, Frere C, Quilici J, Barbou F, Morange PE, Hovasse T, Bonnet J-L, Alessi M-C. High post-treatment platelet reactivity identified low-responders to dual antiplatelet therapy at increased risk of recurrent cardiovascular events after stenting for acute coronary syndrome. J Thromb Haemost 2006; 4: 542-549.

[10]   Chen WH, Lee PY, Ng W, Tse HF, Lau CP. Aspirin resistance is associated with a high incidence of myonecrosis after non-urgent percutaneous coronary intervention despite clopidogrel pretreatment. Am Coll Cardiol 2004; 43: 1122-1126.

[11]   Fitzgerald R, Pirmohamed M. Aspirin resistance: Effect of clinical, biochemical and genetic factors. J. Pharmthera 2011; 130: 213-225.

[12]   Weber AA, Przytulski B, Schanz A, Hohlfeld T, Schrör K. Towards a definition of aspirin resistance: a typological approach. Platelets 2002; 13: 37-40.

[13]   Gum PA, Kottke-Marchant K, Poggio ED, Gurm H, Welsh PA, Brooks L, *et al.* Profile and prevalence of aspirin resistance in patients with cardiovascular disease. Am J Cardiol 2001; 88: 230-5.

[14]   Cañivano Petreñas L, García Yubero C. [Resistance to aspirin: prevalence, mechanisms of action and association with thromboembolic events. A narrative review]. Farm Hosp 2010 Jan-Feb; 34: 32-43.

[15]   Krasopoulos G, Brister SJ, Beattie WS, Buchanan MR. Aspirin "resistance" and risk of cardiovascular morbidity: systematic review and meta-analysis. BMJ 2008; 336: 195-8.

[16]   Aydinalp A, Atar I, Gulmez O, Atar A, Acikel S, Bozbas H, Ozgul A, Ertan C, Ozin B, Muderrisoglu H. The clinical significance of aspirin resistance in patients with chest pain. Clin Cardiol 2010; 33: E1-7.

[17]   Marcucci R, Gori AM, Paniccia R, *et al.* Residual platelet reactivity is associated with clinical and laboratory characteristics in patients with ischaemic heart disease undergoing PCI on dual antiplatelet therapy. Atherosclerosis 2007; 195: 217-23.

[18]   Anfossi G, Russo I, Trovati M. Resistance to aspirin and thienopyridines in diabetes mellitus and metabolic syndrome. Curr Vasc Pharmacol 2008; 6: 313-28.

[19]   Salama MM, Mohamed Morad AR, Saleh MA, Sabri NA, Zaki MM, Elsafady LA. Resistance to low-dose aspirin therapy among patients with acute coronary syndrome in relation to associated risk factors. J Clin Pharm Ther 2012; 37: 630-6.

[20]   Sahin T, Celikyurt U, Geyik B, Oner G, Kilic T, Bildirici U, Kozdag G, Ural D. Relationship Between Endothelial Functions and Acetylsalicylic Acid Resistance in Newly Diagnosed Hypertensive Patients. Clin Cardiol. 2012 Jul 27. doi: 10.1002/clc.22042.

[21]   Valles J., Santos M. T., Fuset M. P., Moscardo A., Ruano M., Perez F., *et al.* Partial inhibition of platelet thromboxane A2 synthesis by aspirin is associated with myonecrosis in patients with ST-segment elevation myocardial infarction. Am J Cardiol 2007; 99; 19-25.

[22]   Kahraman G, Sahin T, Kilic T, Baytugan NZ, Agacdiken A, Ural E, Ural D, Komsuoglu B. The frequency of aspirin resistance and its risk factors in patients with metabolic syndrome. Int J Cardiol 2007; 115: 391-6.

[23]   Alberts MJ, Bergman DL, Molner E, Jovanovic BJ, Ushiwata I, Teruya J. Antiplatelet effect of aspirin in patients with cerebrovascular disease. Stroke. 2004; 35: 175-8.

[24]   Feher G, Koltai K, Papp E, Alkonyi B, Solyom A, Kenyeres P, *et al.* Aspirin resistance: Possible roles of cardiovascular risk factors, previous disease history, concomitant medications and haemorrheological variables. Drugs Aging. 2006; 23: 559-67.

[25]   Lordkipanidzé M, Pharand C, Schampaert E, Turgeon J, Palisaitis DA, Diodati JG. A comparison of six major platelet function tests to determine the prevalence of aspirin resistance in patients with stable coronary artery disease. Eur Heart J 2007; 28: 1702-8.

[26]   Kamath S, Blann AD, Lip GY. Platelet activation: assessment and quantification. Eur Heart J. 2001; 22: 1561-1571.

[27]   Szczeklik A, Musiał J, Undas A, Sanak M. Aspirin resistance. J Thromb Haemost. 2005; 3: 1655-62.

[28]   Mammen EF, Comp PC, Gosselin R. PFA-100TM system: a new method for assessment of platelet dysfunction. Semin Thromb Hemost. 1998; 24: 195-202.

[29]   Michos ED, Ardehali R, Blumenthal RS, Lange RA, Ardehali H. Aspirin and clopidogrel resistance. Mayo Clin Proc 2006; 81: 518-26.

[30]   Perneby C, Granstrom E, Beck O, *et al.* Optimization of an enzyme immunoassay for 11-dehydro-thromboxane B(2) in urine: comparison with GC-MS. Thromb Res 1999; 96: 427-436.

[31]   Faraday N, Becker DM, Yanek LR, *et al.* Relation between atherosclerosis risk factors and aspirin resistance in a primary prevention population. Am J Cardiol 2006; 98: 774-779.

[32]   Grinstein J, Cannon CP. Aspirin Resistance: Current Status and Role of Tailored Therapy. Clin Cardiol. 2012 Jun 27. doi: 10.1002/clc.22031.

[33]   Kuliczkowski W, Witkowski A, Polonski L, Watala C, Filipiak K, Budaj A, Golanski J, *et al.* Interindividual variability in the response to oral antiplatelet drugs: a position paper of the Working Group

on antiplatelet drugs resistance appointed by the Section of Cardiovascular Interventions of the Polish Cardiac Society, endorsed by the Working Group on Thrombosis of the European Society of Cardiology. Eur Heart J 2009; 30: 426-35.

[34]   Neubauer H, Kaiser AF, Endres HG, Krüger JC, Engelhardt A, Lask S, Pepinghege F, Kusber A, Mügge A. Tailored antiplatelet therapy can overcome clopidogrel and aspirin resistance--the BOchum CLopidogrel and Aspirin Plan (BOCLA-Plan) to improve antiplatelet therapy. BMC Med. 2011 Jan 12; 9: 3.

[35]   Berger JS, Bhatt DL, Steg PG, Steinhubl SR, Montalescot G, Shao M, Hacke W, *et al*. Bleeding, mortality, and antiplatelet therapy: results from the Clopidogrel for High Atherothrombotic Risk and Ischemic Stabilization, Management, and Avoidance (CHARISMA) trial. Am Heart J 2011; 162: 98-105.

[36]   Tada T, Natsuaki M, Morimoto T, Furukawa Y, Nakagawa Y, Byrne RA, *et al*.; CREDO-Kyoto PCI/CABG Registry Cohort-2 Investigators. Duration of dual antiplatelet therapy and long-term clinical outcome after coronary drug-eluting stent implantation: landmark analyses from the CREDO-Kyoto PCI/CABG Registry Cohort-2. Circ Cardiovasc Interv 2012; 5: 381-91.

[37]   Gurbel PA, Tantry US. Clopidogrel resistance? Thromb Res 2007; 120: 311-321.

[38]   Uchiyama S. Clopidogrel resistance: identifying and overcoming a barrier to effective antiplatelet treatment. Cardiovasc Ther 2011; 29: e100-11.

[39]   Tantry US, Etherington E, Bilden KP, Gurbel PA. Antiplatelet therapies; current strategies and future trends. Future Cardiol 2006; 2; 343-66.

[40]   Savi P, Herbert JM. Clopidogrel and ticlopidine: P2Y12 adenosine diphosphate-receptor antagonists for the prevention of atherothrombosis. Semin Thromb Hemost 2005; 31: 174-83.

[41]   Hulot JS, Bura A, Villard E, *et al*. Cytochrome P450 2C19 loss-of-function polymorphism is a major determinant of clopidogrel responsiveness in healthy subjects. Blood 2006; 108: 2244-2247.

[42]   Umemura K, Furuta T, Kondo K. The common gene variants of CYP2C19 affect pharmacokinetics and pharmacodynamics in an active metabolite of clopidogrel in healthy subjects. J Thromb Haemost 2008; 6: 1439-1441.

[43]   Gurbel PA, Bliden KP, Hiatt BL, O'Connor CM. Clopidogrel for coronary stenting: response variability, drug resistance, and the effect of pre-treatment platelet reactivity. Circulation 2003; 107: 2908-13.

[44]   Schmidt M, Johansen MB, Maeng M, Kaltoft A, Jensen LO, Tilsted HH, Bøtker HE, *et al*. Concomitant use of clopidogrel and statins and risk of major adverse cardiovascular events following coronary stent implantation. Br J Clin Pharmacol 2012; 74: 161-70.

[45]   Abraham NS, Hlatky MA, Antman EM, Bhatt DL, Bjorkman DJ, Clark CB, Furberg CD, *et al*. ACCF/ACG/AHA 2010 Expert Consensus Document on the concomitant use of proton pump inhibitors and thienopyridines: a focused update of the ACCF/ACG/AHA 2008 expert consensus document on reducing the gastrointestinal risks of antiplatelet therapy and NSAID use: a report of the American College of Cardiology Foundation Task Force on Expert Consensus Documents. Circulation 2010; 122: 2619-2633.

[46]   Nguyen TA, Diodati JG, Pharand C. Resistance to clopidogrel: a review of the evidence. J Am Coll Cardiol. 2005; 45: 1157-1164.

[47]   Lau WC, Gurbel PA, Watkins PB, *et al*. Contribution of hepatic cytochrome P450 3A4 metabolic activity to the phenomenon of clopidogrel resistance. Circulation. 2004; 109: 166-171.

[48]   Taubert D, Kastrati A, Harlfinger S, *et al*. Pharmacokinetics of clopidogrel after administiration of a high loading dose. Thromb Haemost 2004; 92: 311-6.

[49]   Von Beckerath N, Taubert D, Pogatsa-Murray G, *et al*. Absorption, metabolization, and antiplatelet effects of 300-, 600-, 900-mg loading doses of clopidogrel: results of the ISAR-CHOICE trial. Circulation 2005; 112: 2946-50.

[50]   Gori AM, Cesari F, Marcucci R, *et al*. The balance between pro- and anti-inflammatory cytokines is associated with platelet aggregability in acute coronary syndrome patients. Atherosclerosis 2009; 202: 255-62.

[51]   Matetzky S, Shenkman B, Guetta V, *et al*. Clopidogrel resistance is associated with increased risk of recurrent atherothrombotic events in patients with acute myocardial infarction Circulation 2004; 109: 3171-3175.

[52]   Buonamici P, Marcucci R, Migliorini A, Gensini GF, Santini A, Paniccia R, *et al*. Impact of platelet reactivity after clopidogrel administration on drug-eluting stent thrombosis. J Am Coll Cardiol 2007; 49: 2312-2317.

[53]   Soffer D, Moussa I, Harjaim KJ, Boura JA, Dixon SR, Grines CL, *et al.* Impact of angina class on inhibition of platelet aggregation following clopidogrel loading in patients undergoing coronary intervention: Do we need more aggressive dosing regimens in unstable angina? Catheterization and Cardiovascular Interventions 2003; 59: 21-25.

[54]   Pinto Slottow TL, Bonello L, Gavini R, *et al.* Prevalence of aspirin and clopidogrel resistance among patients with and without drug-eluting stent thrombosis. Am J Cardiol 2009; 104: 525-530.

[55]   Blais N, Pharand C, Lordkipanidz´e M, *et al.* Response to aspirin in healthy individuals. Cross comparison of light transmission aggregometry, VerifyNow system, platelet count drop, thromboelastography (TEG) and urinary 11-dehydrothromboxane B(2). Thromb Haemost 2009; 102: 404-411.

[56]   Ganter MT, Hofer CK. Coagulation monitoring: Current techniques and clinical use of viscoelastic point-of-care coagulation devices. Anesth Analg 2008; 106: 1366-1375.

[57]   Lordkipanidz´e M, Pharand C, Schampaert E, *et al.* Evaluation of the platelet count drop method for assessment of platelet function in comparison with "gold standard" light transmission aggregometry. Thromb Res 2009; 124: 418-422.

[58]   Breet NJ, van Werkum JW, Bouman HJ, *et al.* Comparison of platelet function tests in predicting clinical outcome in patients undergoing coronary stent implantation. JAMA 2010; 303: 754-762.

[59]   Gurbel PA, Bliden KP, Hiatt BL, O'Connor CM. Clopidogrel for coronary stenting: response variability, drug resistance, and the effect of pretreatment platelet reactivity. Circulation 2003; 107: 2908-13.

[60]   Gurbel PA, Bliden KP, Hayes KM, Yoho JA, Herzog WR, Tantry US. The relation of dosing to clopidogrel responsiveness and the incidence of high post-treatment platelet aggregation in patients undergoing coronary stenting. J Am Coll Cardiol 2005; 45: 1392-6.

[61]   Mehta SR, Tanguay JF, Eikelboom JW, Jolly SS, Joyner CD, Granger CB, Faxon DP, *et al.* Double-dose *versus* standard-dose clopidogrel and high-dose *versus* low-dose aspirin in individuals undergoing percutaneous coronary intervention for acute coronary syndromes (CURRENT-OASIS 7): a randomised factorial trial. Lancet 2010; 376: 1233-1243.

[62]   Koul S, Smith JG, Schersten F, James S, Lagerqvist B, Erlinge D. Effect of upstream clopidogrel treatment in patients with ST-segment elevation myocardial infarction undergoing primary percutaneous coronary intervention. Eur Heart J 2011; 32: 2989-2997.

[63]   Gurbel PA, Bliden KP, Zaman KA, Yoho JA, Hayes KM, Tantry US. Clopidogrel loading with eptifibatide to arrest the reactivity of platelets: results of the Clopidogrel Loading With Eptifibatide to Arrest the Reactivity of Platelets (CLEAR PLATELETS) study. Circulation 2005; 111: 1153-9.

[64]   Montalescot G, Sideris G, Meuleman C, *et al.* A randomized comparison of high clopidogrel loading-doses in patients with non-ST-elevation acute coronary syndromes: the ALBION trial. J Am Coll Cardiol 2006; 48: 931-938.

[65]   Cuisset T, Quilici J, Cohen W, Fourcade L, Saut N, Pankert M, Gaborit B, *et al.* Usefulness of high clopidogrel maintenance dose according to CYP2C19 genotypes in clopidogrel low responders undergoing coronary stenting for non ST elevation acute coronary syndrome. Am J Cardiol 2011; 108: 760-5.

[66]   Han YL, Wang B, Li Y, Xu K, Wang SL, Jing QM, Wang ZL, *et al.* A high maintenance dose of clopidogrel improves short-term clinical outcomes in patients with acute coronary syndrome undergoing drug-eluting stent implantation. Chin Med J (Engl) 2009; 122: 793-7.

[67]   Aradi D, Rideg O, Vorobcsuk A, Magyarlaki T, Magyari B, Kónyi A, Pintér T, *et al.* Justification of 150 mg clopidogrel in patients with high on-clopidogrel platelet reactivity. Eur J Clin Invest 2012; 42: 384-92.

[68]   Angiolillo DJ, Shoemaker SB, Desai B, Yuan H, Charlton RK, Bernardo E, Zeni MM, *et al.* Randomized comparison of a high clopidogrel maintenance dose in patients with diabetes mellitus and coronary artery disease: results of the Optimizing Antiplatelet Therapy in Diabetes Mellitus (OPTIMUS) study. Circulation 2007; 115: 708-16.

[69]   Sardella G, Calcagno S, Mancone M, Palmirotta R, Lucisano L, Canali E, Stio RE, *et al.* Pharmacodynamic Effect of Switching Therapy in Patients With High On-Treatment Platelet Reactivity and Genotype Variation With High Clopidogrel Dose *Versus* Prasugrel: The RESET GENE Trial. Circ Cardiovasc Interv 2012; 5: 698-704.

[70]   Wiviott SD, Trenk D, Frelinger AL, O'Donoghue M, Neumann FJ, Michelson AD, Angiolillo DJ, *et al*; PRINCIPLE-TIMI 44 Investigators. Prasugrel compared with high loading- and maintenance-dose clopidogrel in patients with planned percutaneous coronary intervention: the Prasugrel in Comparison to

Clopidogrel for Inhibition of Platelet Activation and Aggregation-Thrombolysis in Myocardial Infarction 44 trial. Circulation 2007; 116: 2923-32.

[71]   Montalescot G, Sideris G, Cohen R, Meuleman C, Bal dit Sollier C, Barthélémy O, Henry P, *et al.* Prasugrel compared with high-dose clopidogrel in acute coronary syndrome. The randomised, double-blind ACAPULCO study. Thromb Haemost 2010; 103: 213-23.

[72]   Alexopoulos D, Xanthopoulou I, Davlouros P, Plakomyti TE, Panagiotou A, Mavronasiou E, Hahalis G. Prasugrel overcomes high on-clopidogrel platelet reactivity in chronic coronary artery disease patients more effectively than high dose (150 mg) clopidogrel. Am Heart J 2011; 162: 733-9.

[73]   Angiolillo DJ, Badimon JJ, Saucedo JF, Frelinger AL, Michelson AD, Jakubowski JA, Zhu B, *et al.* A pharmacodynamic comparison of prasugrel *vs.* high-dose clopidogrel in patients with type 2 diabetes mellitus and coronary artery disease: results of the Optimizing anti-Platelet Therapy In diabetes MellitUS (OPTIMUS)-3 Trial. Eur Heart J 2011; 32: 838-46.

[74]   Steiner S, Moertl D, Chen L, Coyle D, Wells GA. Network meta-analysis of prasugrel, ticagrelor, high- and standard-dose clopidogrel in patients scheduled for percutaneous coronary interventions. Thromb Haemost 2012; 108: 318-27.

[75]   Jeong YH, Hwang JY, Kim IS, Park Y, Hwang SJ, Lee SW, Kwak CH, Park SW. Adding cilostazol to dual antiplatelet therapy achieves greater platelet inhibition than high maintenance dose clopidogrel in patients with acute myocardial infarction: Results of the adjunctive cilostazol *versus* high maintenance dose clopidogrel in patients with AMI (ACCEL-AMI) study. Circ Cardiovasc Interv 2010; 3: 17-26.

[76]   Hu T, Ma H, Li H, Ren J. Efficacy of Cilostazol in Patients With Acute Coronary Syndrome After Percutaneous Coronary Intervention. Am J Ther. 2012 Sep 12. [Epub ahead of print]

[77]   Jeong YH, Lee SW, Choi BR, *et al.* Randomized comparison of adjunctive cilostazol *versus* high maintenance dose clopidogrel in patients with high post-treatment platelet reactivity: Results of the ACCEL-RESISTANCE (Adjunctive Cilostazol *Versus* High Maintenance Dose Clopidogrel in Patients With Clopidogrel Resistance) randomized study. J Am Coll Cardiol 2009; 53: 1101-1109.

[78]   Shim CY, Yoon SJ, Park S, *et al.* The clopidogrel resistance can be attenuated with triple antiplatelet therapy in patients undergoing drug-eluting stents implantation. Int J Cardiol 2009; 134: 351-355.

[79]   Steinhubl SR, Talley JD, Braden GA, Tcheng JE, Casterella PJ, Moliterno DJ, Navetta FI, Berger PB, Popma JJ, Dangas G, Gallo R, Sane DC, Saucedo JF, Jia G, Lincoff AM, Theroux P, Holmes DR, Teirstein PS, Kereiakes DJ. Point-of-care measured platelet inhibition correlates with a reduced risk of an adverse cardiac event after percutaneous coronary intervention: results of the GOLD (AU-Assessing Ultegra) multicenter study. Circulation 2001; 103: 2572-2578.

CHAPTER 6

Platelet Inhibitors for the Treatment of Acute Coronary Syndromes

Hasan Gungor[*] and Ceyhun Ceyhan

Department of Cardiology, Adnan Menderes University, Aydın, Turkey

Abstract: Acute coronary syndrome (ACS) is associated with significant morbidity, mortality and it is a major public health problem. The primary pathophysiological mechanism of the ACS is the response to vascular injury such as atherosclerotic plaque rupture or endothelial monolayer erosion that triggers platelet activation and aggregation leading to platelet-rich thrombi. These platelet-rich thrombi impair blood flow and result in ischemia. Inhibition of platelet aggregation by medical treatment prevents formation and progression of thrombotic process. Antiplatelet therapy is indispensible in the early and long-term management of patients with ACS. Current platelet inhibitors are thromboxane inhibitors (aspirin), P2Y12 inhibitors (ticlopidine, clopidogrel, prasugrel, ticagrelor, cangrelor and elinogrel) and protease-activated receptor antagonists (vorapaxar and atopaxar). The aim of this chapter is to discuss anti platelet therapy in ACS.

Keywords: Acute coronary syndrome, antiplatelet therapy, aspirin, atherosclerosis, atoxapar, cangrelor, coronary artery disease, clopidogrel, elinogrel, inflammation, irreversible, platelets, prasugrel, protease-activated receptor, reversible, thienopyridine, thrombosis, thromboxane, ticagrelor, voraxapar.

INTRODUCTION

Acute coronary syndrome (ACS) is associated with significant morbidity, mortality and it is a major public health problem [1]. Each year in the United States of America, 1300000 patients are admitted to the hospital with ACS. Worldwide 7 million people each year are estimated to have ST segment elevation myocardial infarction (STEMI) and non-ST segment elevation myocardial infarction (NSTEMI) [2].

The primary pathophysiological mechanism of the ACS is the platelet-rich thrombi formation developing in response to vascular injury such as atherosclerotic plaque rupture or endothelial monolayer erosion.

---

*Corresponding author Hasan Gungor: Department of Cardiology, Adnan Menderes University, Aydın, Turkey; E-mail: drgungorhasan@yahoo.com

Ertugrul Ercan and Gulfem Ece (Eds.)

Atherosclerotic plaque rupture or endothelial monolayer erosion triggers platelet activation and aggregation, leading to platelet-rich thrombi. These platelet-rich thrombi impair blood flow and result in ischemia.

Compared with red cell thrombi, platelet-rich thrombi are difficult to lyse and promote development of acute reocclusion [3].

Inhibition of platelet aggregation by medical treatment prevents formation and progression of thrombotic processes (Fig. **1**). These treatment modalities are important for the prevention of complication after ACS. Antiplatelet therapy is indispensible in the early and long-term management of patients with ACS [4].

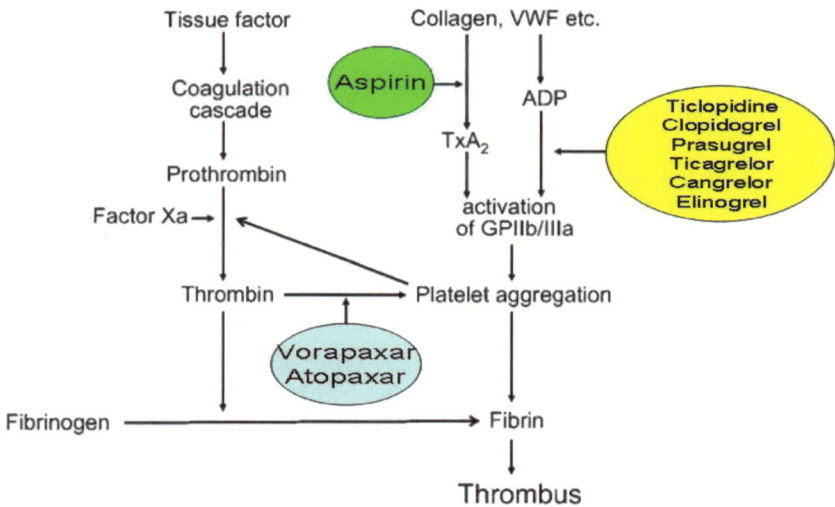

Figure 1: The coagulation cascade.

Current platelet inhibitors are thromboxane inhibitors (aspirin), P2Y12 inhibitors (ticlopidine, clopidogrel, prasugrel, ticagrelor, cangrelor and elinogrel) and protease-activated receptor antagonists (vorapaxar and atopaxar) [5] (Table **1**). The aim of this chapter is to discuss antiplatelet treatment in ACS patients.

Thromboxane A2 Inhibitors

Aspirin

Aspirin irreversibly inhibits COX-1 by acetylating serine 529 and the production of TxA2. For over 50 years, aspirin has been mainstay of antiplatelet therapy in patients with ACS [3]. The efficacy of aspirin for the primary treatment of ACS patients and secondary prevention has been shown in clinical trials and meta-analyses [6, 7]. In high risk patients with ACS, aspirin reduces vascular death by 15% and non-fatal vascular events by 30% [8]. However morbidity, mortality and bleeding risk remain higher with aspirin. Despite its wide use, the optimal effective and safe treatment dose of aspirin is unclear. Recent studies have suggested that 300 mg aspirin is similar to 75-100 mg aspirin for the prevention of vascular events [6].

Table 1: Summary of antiplatelet agents

Drug	Class	Administration	Metabolism	Reversibility	Frequency	Approved	Limitation
Aspirin	TxA2 inhibitor	Oral	Direct acting	Irreversible	Daily	1988	Weak
Ticlopidine	Thienopyridine	Oral	CYP-450 mediated	Irreversible	Twice daily	1991	More side effect
Clopidogrel	Thienopyridine	Oral	CYP-450 mediated	Irreversible	Daily	1997	Variable response
Prasugrel	Thienopyridine	Oral	CYP-450 mediated	Irreversible	Daily	2009	Higher-risk of bleeding
Ticagrelor	Cyclopentyltri-azolopyrimidine	Oral	Not a pro-drug	Reversible	Twice daily	2010	Dyspnea and ventricular pauses
Cangrelor	Non-thienopyridine	Intravenous	Not a pro-drug	Reversible	-	Not approved	Higher risk of bleeding
Elinogrel	Non-thienopyridine	Intravenous and oral	Not a pro-drug	Reversible	-	Not approved	?
Vorapaxar	Trycylic 3-phenylpridine	Oral	Not a pro-drug	Reversible	Daily	Not approved	Bleeding
Atoxapar	-	Oral	Not a pro-drug	Reversible	Daily	Not approved	Bleeding

CURRENT-OASIS 7 trial compared the higher dose aspirin ($\geq$300 mg/day) with low dose (75-81 mg/day) in ACS patients and demonstrated similar end-points with the risk of major bleeding complications [9].

According to the ACC/AHA 2011 guidelines on UA/NSTEMI and ESC 2011 guidelines on UA/NSTEMI, a loading dose of 162-325 mg (or 250-500 mg bolus intravenous) and 75-162 mg/day following dose should be given indefinitely unless active bleeding or allergy [10, 11].

Aspirin acts by irreversibly inhibiting platelet COX-1 and this effect is reversed when new unaffected platelets enter the circulation after 7 to 14 days. A proton pump inhibitor should also be added to the patients with gastrointestinal bleeding or duodenal ulcer. However aspirin only blocks the TxA2 cascade, platelet activation and platelet-rich thrombi *via* other pathways may occur.

P2Y12 Inhibitors

P2Y12 inhibitors include ticlopidine, clopidogrel, prasugrel and ticagrelor. Ticlopidine, clopidogrel and prasugrel are three generations of thienopyridines that irreversibly and selectively inhibit the P2Y12 receptors.

Ticlopidine

Ticlopidine is the first-generation and first approved thienopyridine that requires metabolism by the hepatic cytochrome P450-1A enzyme system [12]. It is rapidly absorbed and metabolized after twice a day oral administration. The bioavailability of this drug is increased by food and decreased by antacids. Ticlopidine Aspirin Stroke Study showed that ticlopidine was superior to aspirin for non-fatal stroke or death [13]. However there have only been few studies that examined ticlopidine in unstable angina.

Ticlopidine showed 6.3% reduction in combined end point of vascular death and non-fatal myocardial infarction compared with no antiplatelet therapy [14]. This drug also showed similar outcomes with aspirin in UAP patients [8].

Ticlopidine has several limitations such as neutropenia, thrombotic thrombocytopenic purpura and rash. Diarrhea, nausea and vomiting occur in 30% to 50% of ticlopidine recipient patients. Neutropenia is the most serious side effect and can be seen in 2.1% of patients. Blood counts should be performed two or three weeks during the first 3 months of treatment [15]. Ticlopidine has been largely replaced by clopidogrel in patients with atheroslerotic cardiovascular disease.

Clopidogrel

Clopidogrel is a second generation thienopyridine and it is metabolized by the hepatic cytochrome P450 system in the liver. Before intestinal absorption, 85% of the pro-drug is hydrolyzed by esterases to an inactive carboxylic acid derivate and several hours are required to reach therapeutic levels.

The first clinical evidence of clopidogrel in ACS patients is the presence of Clopidogrel in Unstable Angina to Prevent Recurrent Events (CURE) and the substudy of PCI-CURE trials [16, 17]. In CURE trial, a total of 12562 patients with NSTE-ACS followed for 12 months receiving placebo or clopidogrel in addition to aspirin. Clopidogrel treatment significantly reduced primary endpoint of MI, death or stroke (Fig. **2**). Clopidogrel was associated with an increase in major bleeding complications.

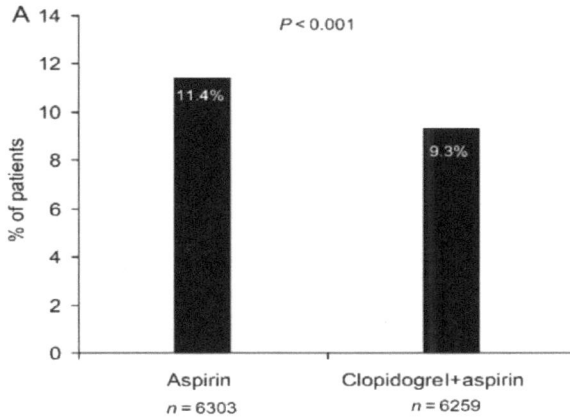

Figure 2: Clopidogrel treatment significantly reduced primary endpoint of MI, death or stroke.

Also in PCI-CURE trial, patients undergoing PCI who were pretreated with clopidogrel had a significantly lower rate of primary endpoint with 30 days of PCI. These findings demonstrated that the clopidogrel with aspirin reduces risk of major adverse cardiac events in ACS patients.

The COMMIT (Clopidogrel and Metoprolol in Myocardial Infarction Trial) and the CLARITY (Clopidogrel as Adjunctive Reperfusion Therapy-Thrombolysis in Myocardial Infarction) trial showed the benefit of dual antiplatelet therapy in patients with STEMI. In COMMIT trial, 45852 patients with STEMI followed with aspirin treatment also received either clopidogrel 75 mg or placebo for up to 4 weeks. Composite endpoint of reinfarction, death, or stroke were significantly lower in patients receiving clopidogrel plus aspirin *versus* those receiving aspirin alone. A significant reduction in all-cause death (co-primary endpoint) was also detected with clopidogrel plus aspirin [18].

In CLARITY trial, 3491 patients with STEMI treated with aspirin and fibrinolytic therapy were randomized to receive either clopidogrel (300 mg loading dose followed by 75 mg/day) or placebo. The incidence of the primary efficacy endpoint (composite of an occluded infarct-related artery on angiography or death or recurrent MI before angiography) was significantly reduced in the clopidogrel plus aspirin group *versus* aspirin [19].

The CAPRIE (Clopidogrel *versus* Aspirin in Patients at Risk of Ischemic Events) trial evaluated the efficacy of clopidogrel 75 mg *versus* aspirin 325 mg in secondary prevention of atherothrombotic disease in 19185 patients with prior MI, stroke/TIA, or symptomatic PAD. The incidence of the primary composite endpoint of ischemic stroke, MI, and vascular death was 5.3% in the clopidogrel group and 5.8% in the aspirin group [20].

The CURRENT-OASIS 7 (Clopidogrel Optimal Loading Dose Usage to Reduce Recurrent Events/Optimal Antiplatelet Strategy for Interventions) trial evaluated the effect of standard (300 mg loading dose plus 75 mg once daily maintenance dose) and higher-dosing regimens (600 mg loading dose plus 150 mg maintenance dose for 7 days followed by 75 mg maintenance dose) of clopidogrel and aspirin (high-dose regimen of 300-325 mg and standard-dose regimen of 75-100 mg) on cardiovascular outcomes and bleeding complications in 25087 patients with ACS. No significant difference in incidence of the primary composite endpoint of cardiovascular death, MI, or stroke at Day 30 was observed in the overall patient population between the two clopidogrel treatment–groups. However, treatment with high-dose clopidogrel resulted in a significant reduction in the incidence of cardiovascular events *versus* standard-dose clopidogrel in patients who underwent PCI, with a significant reduction in the incidence of MI [21].

On the basis of these findings addition of clopidogrel to aspirin has become the standard therapy in ACS patients. Clopidogrel with loading dose 300-600 mg per oral followed by 75 mg/day is recommended by the ACC/AHA 2011 guidelines on UA/NSTEMI and ESC 2011 guidelines on UA/NSTEMI [10, 11]. A higher dose of 150 mg/daily may be used for the first 7 days in patients who have had a loading dose for PCI.

Despite the fact that aspirin with clopidogrel therapy resulted in a significant benefit, this therapy has several limitations. The residual morbidity and mortality in patients treated with aspirin plus clopidogrel remain high, and the risk of bleeding is increased. Several factors may influence the response to clopidogrel such as poor compliance, drug-drug interactions involving the cytochrome P450 system, genetic polymorphisms and cellular factors.

Suboptimal response to clopidogrel treatment is associated with ischemia or stent thrombosis. This suboptimal response can be attributed to the variation in the CYP gene. This gene codes for the CYP-450 enzymes involved in the biotransformation of the clopidogrel to the active form [22]. Other genetic variations, such as the ABCB1 3435 TT genotype may affect the efficacy of clopidogrel. There is insufficient evidence to test the genetic or platelet function. Higher loading and maintenance doses of clopidogrel are the alternatives in high-risk patients with low responses. Drug-drug interaction is also considered as a cause of clopidogrel suboptimal response. Omeprazole and lansoprazole are proton-pump inhibitors that also inhibit the CYP2C19. If necessary, pantoprazole should be used to diminish side effects [23]. In order the overcome the delayed onset of action and variable inhibition of platelet with clopidogrel, novel antiplatelet treatments have been developed.

Prasugrel

Prasugrel is a third generation thienopyridine and it was approved in 2009 in both Europe and USA. Prasugrel is characterized by the faster onset of action and more effective inhibition of platelet aggregation as compared with clopidogrel [24].

Prasugrel is rapidly hydrolyzed in gastrointestinal system into an intermediary metabolite and this metabolite is hepatically activated. The active metabolite of prasugrel reaches to the peak concentration after 30 minutes and the final concentration is linearly dependent on the prasugrel dose [25]. 70% platelet inhibition is usually achieved within 2-4 hours [26]. Activation of prasugrel involves single CYP-dependent step compared with clopidogrel. Genetic CYP variants do not have clinically significant influence on the active metabolites of prasugrel [24] (Fig. **3**).

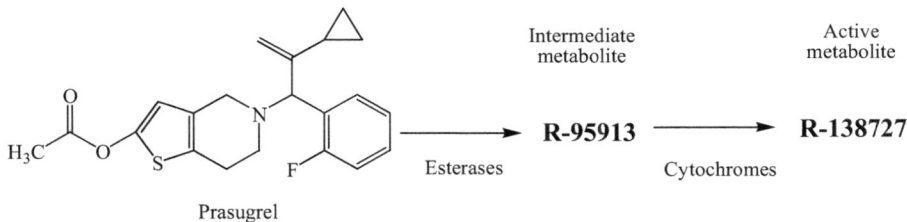

Figure 3: Metabolic pathways of prasugrel.

In PRINCIPLE-TIMI 44 (Prasugrel in Comparison to Clopidogrel for Inhibition of Platelet Activation and Aggregation-Thrombolysis in Myocardial Infarction 44) trial evaluating 201 patients undergoing PCI, loading with 60 mg prasugrel as opposed to 600 mg clopidogrel showed greater and faster inhibition of platelet aggregation with 20 μmol/L ADP at six hours and this difference was evident as early as at 30 minutes. Also inhibition of platelet aggregation after 14 ± 2 days of treatment was higher in patients receiving prasugrel than those receiving clopidogrel [27].

The TRİTON-TIMI (Trial to Assess Improvement in Therapeutic Outcomes by Optimizing Platelet Inhibition with Prasugrel-TIMI) 38 trial, evaluated the efficacy and safety of the combination of prasugrel plus aspirin in patients with ACS. In this trial, 13608 patients with ACS were randomized to prasugrel with 60 mg loading dose and 10 mg daily maintenance dose or clopidogrel with 300 mg loading dose and 75 mg daily maintenance dose. The use of prasugrel was associated with a reduction of cardiovascular death, non-fatal MI or non-fatal stroke. However, the reduction in ischemic end-points with prasugrel was accompanied by a higher incidence of TIMI defined major bleeding, 2.4% *vs.* 1.8% in the prasugrel group [28]. These results suggest that the selection of a P2Y12 ADP receptor antagonist should take into account only the greater pharmacological potency of prasugrel *versus* clopidogrel but also the increased risk for bleeding with prasugrel compared with clopidogrel [29].

For prasugrel there is class II A, level B recommendation. Prasugrel can be used in a 60 mg loading dose followed by 10 mg/daily or 5 mg if the patient weighs < 60 kg. It is not recommended in patients aged >75 years or in patients referred for CABG and it is also contraindicated in patients with a history of transient ischemic attack or stroke.

Ticagrelor

Ticagrelor (AZD6140) is the first oral agent in a new chemical class of nonthienopyridine antiplatelet agents named cyclopentyl-triazolo-pyrimidines. Ticagrelor binds directly and reversibly to P2Y12 without requiring metabolic activation [30]. It was approved in 2010 in USA and Europe. Like prasugrel, ticagrelor acts more rapidly and it is a more potent inhibitor of platelets than clopidogrel without increased major bleedings [31]. Ticagrelor needs 1.5-3.0 hours to reach peak plasma concentrations. Its half life is approximately 12 hours and its antiplatelet effect is low at 48 hours after the last dose [30].

The safety, tolerability and efficacy of this drug were shown in the DISPERSE-2 (Dose confirmation study assessing anti-platelet effects of AZD6140 *vs.* clopidogrel in Non-ST segment elevation myocardial infarction phase II trial). A total of 990 patients with ACS were randomized to 90 or 180 mg ticagrelor twice a day or a clopidogrel 300 mg loading dose plus 75 mg/daily for up to 12 weeks. At 4-week follow-up no difference was observed in major bleeding [32].

Ticagrelor was compared with clopidogrel in PLATO (Study of Platelet Inhibition and Patient Outcomes) trial with 18624 ACS patient [33]. After randomization, the patients received 180 mg loading dose, 90 mg twice daily ticagrelor or 300-600 mg loading dose, 75 mg daily clopidogrel. The primary efficacy endpoint was time to first occurrence of death from vascular causes, MI or stroke. Ticagrelor showed superiority to clopidogrel in reducing rates of the primary endpoint at 12 months (9.8% *vs.* 11.7%, p < 0.001) (Fig. **4**).

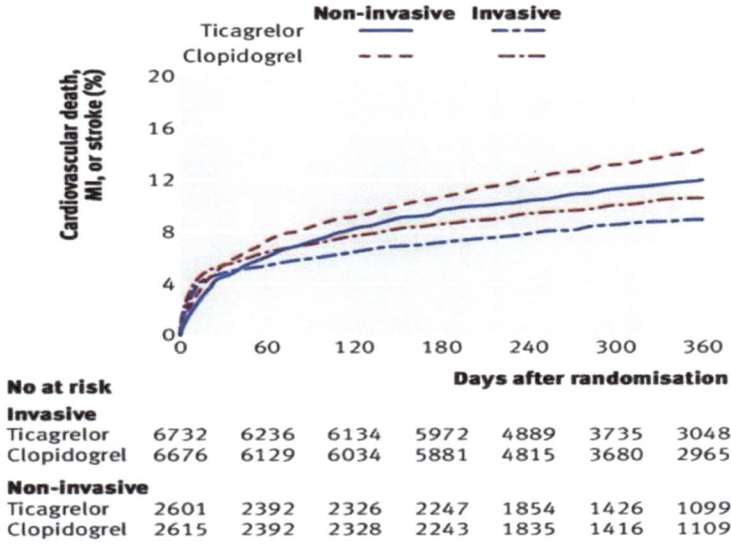

Figure 4: Cumulative incidence of primary composite of cardiovascular death, myocardial infarction and stroke in PLATO trial.

There was also significant reduction in the rate of individual endpoints including all-cause death, cardiovascular death and MI. Major bleeding rate was similar in both groups (11.6% *vs.* 11.2%, p=0.43). Ventricular pauses, mostly in the acute phase of ACS due to the sinus node suppression and mild dyspnea without any adverse effect on cardiac or pulmonary function may be seen to be adenosine-mediates [34].

According to current guidelines, ticagrelor is given as a loading dose of 180 mg per oral, followed by 90 mg twice daily.

Cangrelor

Cangrelor is a reversible, potent, short-acting P2Y12 inhibitor which doer not require metabolic conversion. Unlike the orally-administered other P2Y12 inhibitors, cangrelor is administered by intravenous infusion and it rapidly achieves near complete inhibition of P2Y12 receptors [35].

Cangrelor reaches its steady state concentration in plasma within 30 minutes and it is rapidly cleared from the plasma with 3-5 minutes half-time [36]. Cangrelor is currently evaluated in two-large randomized trials: CHAMPION-PLATFORM and CHAMPION-PCI.

In CHAMPION-PLATFORM trial 5362 patients who had not been treated with clopidogrel to receive either cangrelor or placebo at the time of PCI followed 600 mg clopidogrel. The use periprocedural cangrelor during PCI was not superior to placebo. Major bleeding rate was significantly higher in cangrelor group (3.4% *vs.* 5.4%, p < 0.001) (Fig. **5**) [37].

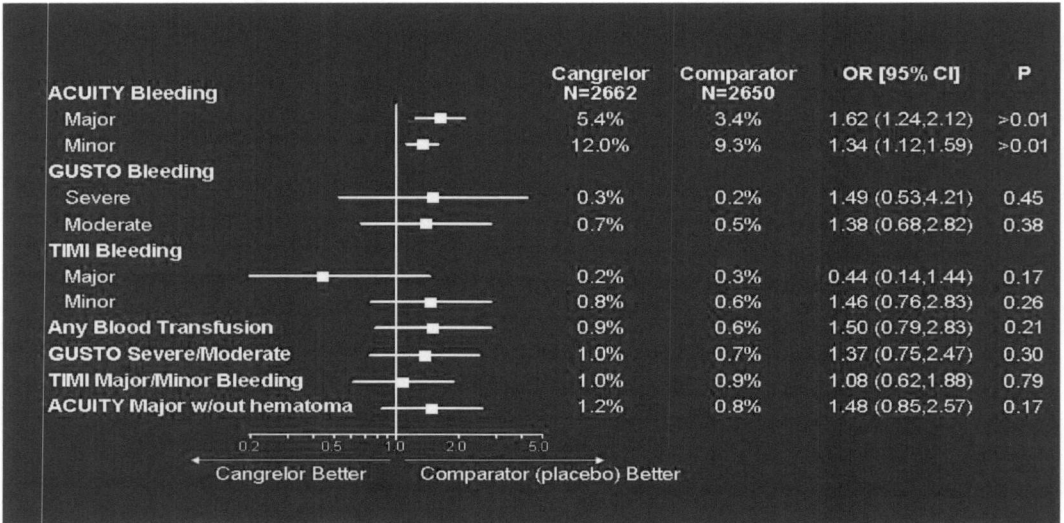

	Cangrelor N=2662	Comparator N=2650	OR [95% CI]	P
ACUITY Bleeding				
Major	5.4%	3.4%	1.62 (1.24,2.12)	>0.01
Minor	12.0%	9.3%	1.34 (1.12,1.59)	>0.01
GUSTO Bleeding				
Severe	0.3%	0.2%	1.49 (0.53,4.21)	0.45
Moderate	0.7%	0.5%	1.38 (0.68,2.82)	0.38
TIMI Bleeding				
Major	0.2%	0.3%	0.44 (0.14,1.44)	0.17
Minor	0.8%	0.6%	1.46 (0.76,2.83)	0.26
Any Blood Transfusion	0.9%	0.6%	1.50 (0.79,2.83)	0.21
GUSTO Severe/Moderate	1.0%	0.7%	1.37 (0.75,2.47)	0.30
TIMI Major/Minor Bleeding	1.0%	0.9%	1.08 (0.62,1.88)	0.79
ACUITY Major w/out hematoma	1.2%	0.8%	1.48 (0.85,2.57)	0.17

Cangrelor Better ← → Comparator (placebo) Better

Figure 5: Bleeding rates from CHAMPION-PLATFORM trial.

In CHAMPION-PCI trial 8716 patients compared 600 mg oral clopidogrel treatment with cangrelor before PCI in ACS patients. Cangrelor was administered intravenously 30 minutes before PCI and continued for 2 hours after PCI. Cangrelor treatment was not superior to clopidogrel [38]. In May 2009, both trials have been stopped following a decision by the interim analysis review committee.

Like cangrelor, elinogrel is a direct-acting reversible P2Y12 receptor inhibitor that is in phase 2 clinical trial. Elinogrel is administered both intravenously and orally, it is is not requiring metabolic conversion. In preclinical studies, elinogrel showed antithrombotic activity *in vivo* plasma concentrations with minimal bleeding rate [39]. Phase 3 investigations are currently being designed.

Protease-Activated Receptor Antagonists

Protease-activated receptor antagonists (PARs) include PAR1, PAR2, PAR3, PAR4 and in human platelets, only PAR1 and PAR4 are expressed. The PARs are G protein-coupled receptors that mediate the cellular effects of different proteases like thrombin [40, 41]. The PARs have well-known role in homeostasis, atherothrombosis and vascular biology [40]. PAR1-mediated platelet activation promotes pathological thrombosis with less influence on protective homeostasis. PAR1 antagonists decrease the incidence of haemorrhagic complications [42, 43]. Two PAR1 antagonists are currently being researched include vorapaxar and atopaxar.

Vorapaxar

Vorapaxar is a synthetic tricylic 3-phenylpyridine and it is orally active fourth generation himbacine based antagonist of the PAR1. Vorapaxar is a non-peptide competitive PAR1 antagonist with low molecular weight and high affinity [42]. Vorapaxar inhibits thrombin-mediated platelet aggregation without increasing bleeding time. It is rapidly absorbed and has a long biological half-life [44, 45]. Vorapaxar has shown to completely inhibit PAR1 induced platelet aggregation with oral administration in animal models with 86% bioavailability [46].

The Thrombin Receptor Antagonist for Clinical Event Reduction in ACS (TRACER) and Thrombin Receptor Antagonist in Secondary Prevention of Atherothrombotic Ischaemic Events (TRA 2P-TIMI 50) trials have been designed to evaluate the reduction of recurrent ischaemic events with vorapaxar [47, 48].

The TRACER trial is designed to assess whether the vorapaxar added to aspirin plus clopidogrel will reduce the incidence of cardiovascular death, MI, stroke, recurrent ischaemia and urgent revascularization in ACS patients. A total of 10000 patients will evaluate with 40 mg loading dose and 2.5 mg daily maintaining dose of vorapaxar for at least 1 year *versus* placebo [47].

In the TRA 2P-TIMI 50 trial 2.5 mg daily maintenance dose of vorapaxar *versus* placebo in addition to current standard therapy. The study has completed enrollment of approximately 26000 patients. The primary end-point of this trial is the composite of the first occurrence of any cardiovascular death, MI, stroke and urgent coronary revascularization during 1 year follow-up [48].

Subgroup analysis of TRA 2P-TIMI 50 trial showed that at 3 years, the primary end point had occurred in 1028 patients (9.3%) in the vorapaxar group and in

1176 patients (10.5%) in the placebo group (hazard ratio for the vorapaxar group, 0.87; 95% confidence interval [CI], 0.80 to 0.94; P < 0.001). Cardiovascular death, myocardial infarction, stroke, or recurrent ischemia leading to revascularization occurred in 1259 patients (11.2%) in the vorapaxar group and 1417 patients (12.4%) in the placebo group (hazard ratio, 0.88; 95% CI, 0.82 to 0.95; P=0.001). Moderate or severe bleeding occurred in 4.2% of patients who received vorapaxar and 2.5% of those who received placebo (hazard ratio, 1.66; 95% CI, 1.43 to 1.93; P < 0.001) (Fig. **6**). There was an increase in the rate of intracranial hemorrhage in the vorapaxar group (1.0%, *vs.* 0.5% in the placebo group; P < 0.001) [49].

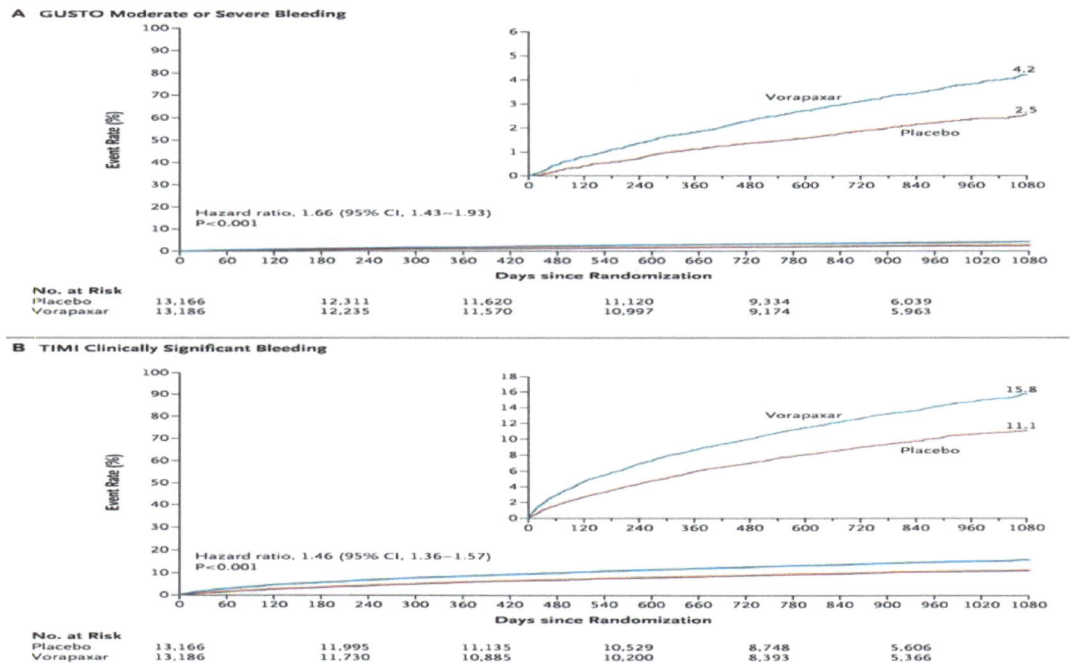

Figure 6: Moderate or severe bleeding rate was significantly higher in vorapaxar group.

CONCLUSION

New P2Y12 inhibitors have decreased ischemic events after ACS compared with clopidogrel. Despite the-improvements in clinical outcomes with the new P12Y12 inhibitors, remaining questions are the duration of therapy, different doses, drug-drug interactions, cost effectiveness and optimal time of initiation in ACS patients. Current clinical practice guidelines recommend 12 months treatment with dual antiplatelet therapy in patients with ACS. However, residual morbidity and mortality remain substantial even in these patients. New antiplatelet agents with a more favorable benefit-to-risk profile should be investigated in future trials.

ACKNOWLEDGEMENTS

Declared none.

CONFLICT OF INTEREST

The authors confirm that this chapter contents have no conflict of interest.

REFERENCES

[1]   Van de Werf F. New antithrombotic agents: are they needed and what can they offer to patients with a non-ST-elevation acute coronary syndrome? Eur Heart J 2009; 30: 1695-702.
[2]   Lloyd-Jones D, Adams RJ, Brown TM, *et al*. Heart disease and stroke statistics-2010 update: a report from the American Heart Association. Circulation. 2010; 121: e46-e215.
[3]   Boersma E, Harrington RA, Moliterno DJ, *et al*. Platelet glycoprotein IIb/IIIa inhibitors in acute coronary syndromes: a meta-analysis of all major randomised clinical trials. Lancet 2002; 359: 189-98.
[4]   Wijns W, Kolh P, Danchin N, Di Mario C, Falk V, Folliguet T, Garg S, Huber K, James S, Knuuti J, Lopez-Sendon J, Marco J, Menicanti L, Ostojic M, Piepoli MF, Pirlet C, Pomar JL, Reifart N, Ribichini FL, Schalij MJ, Sergeant P, Serruys PW, Silber S, Sousa Uva M, Taggart D. Guidelines on myocardial revascularization: The Task Force on Myocardial Revascularization of the European Society of Cardiology (ESC) and the European Association for Cardio-Thoracic Surgery (EACTS). Eur Heart J 2010; 31: 2501-5.
[5]   Meadows TA, Bhatt DL. Clinical aspects of platelet inhibitors and thrombus formation. Circ Res 2007; 100: 1261-75.
[6]   Antithrombotic Trialists' (ATT) Collaboration, Baigent C, Blackwell L, Collins R, Emberson J, Godwin J, Peto R, Buring J, Hennekens C, Kearney P, Meade T, Patrono C, Roncaglioni MC, Zanchetti A: Aspirin in the primary and secondary prevention of vascular disease: collaborative meta-analysis of individual participant data from randomised trials. Lancet 2009; 373: 1849-60.
[7]   Cairns JA, Gent M, Singer J, Finnie KJ, Froggatt GM, Holder DA, Jablonsky G, Kostuk WJ, Melendez LJ, Myers MG. Aspirin, sulfinpyrazone, or both in unstable angina. Results of a Canadian multicenter trial. N Engl J Med 1985; 313: 1369-75.
[8]   Antithrombotic Trialists' Collaboration. Collaborative metaanalysis of randomised trials of antiplatelet therapy for prevention of death, myocardial infarction, and stroke in high risk patients. BMJ 2002; 324: 71-86.
[9]   CURRENT-OASIS 7 Investigators, Mehta SR, Bassand JP, Chrolavicius S, Diaz R, Eikelboom JW, Fox KA, Granger CB, Jolly S, Joyner CD, Rupprecht HJ, Widimsky P, Afzal R, Pogue J, Yusuf S: Dose comparisons of clopidogrel and aspirin in acute coronary syndromes. N Engl J Med 2010; 363: 930-42.
[10]   ACCF/AHA Focused update of the guidelines for the management of patients with unstable angina/non-ST-elevation myocardial infarction (Updating the 2007 Guideline). J Am Coll Cardiol. 2011; 57: 1920-59.
[11]   ESC Guidelines for the management of acute coronary sydromes in patients presenting without persistent ST-segment elevation. Eur Heart J 2011; 32: 2999-3054.
[12]   Varga-Szabo D, Pleines I, Nieswandt B: Cell adhesion mechanisms in platelets. Arterioscler Thromb Vasc Biol 2008; 28: 403-12.

[13] Hass WK, Easton JD, Adam HP, Pryse-Phillips W, Molony BA, Anderson S, Kamm B, and the Ticlopidine Aspirin Stroke Study Group: A Randomized Trial Comparing Ticlopidine Hydrochloride with Aspirin for the Prevention of Stroke in High-Risk Patients. N Engl J Med, 1989; 321: 501-7.

[14] Balsano F, Violi F, Cimminiello C. Ticlopidine in unstable angina. Circulation 1990; 82: 2282-83.

[15] Gent M, Blakely JA, Easton JD, Ellis DJ, Hachinski VC, Harbison JW, Panak E, Roberts RS, Sicurella J, Turpie AG. The Canadian American Ticlopidine Study (CATS) in thromboembolic stroke. Lancet 1989; 1: 1215-20.

[16] Peters RJ, Mehta SR, Fox KA, Zhao F, Lewis BS, Kopecky SL, Diaz R, Commerford PJ, Valentin V, Yusuf S; Clopidogrel in Unstable angina to prevent Recurrent Events (CURE) Trial Investigators. Effects of aspirin dose when used alone or in combination with clopidogrel in patients with acute coronary syndromes: observations from the Clopidogrel in Unstable angina to preventRecurrent Events (CURE) study. Circulation 2003; 108: 1682-87.

[17] Mehta SR, Yusuf S, Peters RJ, Bertrand ME, Lewis BS, Natarajan MK, Malmberg K, Rupprecht H, Zhao F, Chrolavicius S, Copland I, Fox KA; Clopidogrel in Unstable angina to prevent Recurrent Events trial (CURE) Investigators. Effects of pretreatment with clopidogrel and aspirin followed by long-term therapy in patients undergoing percutaneous coronary intervention: the PCI-CURE study. Lancet 2001; 358: 527-33.

[18] Chen ZM, Jiang LX, Chen YP, Xie JX, Pan HC, Peto R, Collins R, Liu LS. Addition of clopidogrel to aspirin in 45,852 patients with acute myocardial infarction: randomised placebo-controlled trial. Lancet 2005; 366: 1607-21.

[19] Sabatine MS, Cannon CP, Gibson CM, López-Sendón JL, Montalescot G, Theroux P, Claeys MJ, Cools F, Hill KA, Skene AM, McCabe CH, Braunwald E. Addition of clopidogrel to aspirin and fibrinolytic therapy for myocardial infarction with STsegment elevation. N Engl J Med 2005; 352: 1179-89.

[20] CAPRIE Steering Commitee. A randomised, blinded, trial of clopidogrel versus aspirin in patients at risk of ischaemic events (CAPRIE). CAPRIE Steering Committee. Lancet 1996; 348: 1329-39.

[21] Mehta SR, Bassand JP, Chrolavicius S, Diaz R, Fox KA, Granger CB, Jolly S, Rupprecht HJ, Widimsky P, Yusuf S. Design and rationale of CURRENT-OASIS 7: a randomized, 2x2 factorial trial evaluating optimal dosing strategies for clopidogrel and aspirin in patients with ST and non-ST-elevation acute coronary syndromes managed with an early invasive strategy. Am Heart J 2008; 156: 1080-88.

[22] Farid NA, Kurihara A, Wrighton SA. Metabolism and disposition of the thienopyridine antiplatelet drugs ticlopidine, clopidogrel, and prasugrel in humans. J Clin Pharmacol 2010; 50: 126-142.

[23] Stockl KM, Le L, Zakharyan A, Solow BK, Addiego JE, Ramsey S. Risk of rehospitalization for patients using clopidogrel with a proton pump inhibitor. Arch Intern Med 2010; 170: 704-10.

[24] Jernberg T, Payne CD, Winters KJ, Darstein C, Brandt JT, Jakubowski JA, Naganuma H, Siegbahn A, Wallentin L. Prasugrel achieves greater inhibition of platelet aggregation and a lower rate of non-responders compared with clopidogrel in aspirin-treated patients with stable coronary artery disease. Eur Heart J 2006; 27: 1166-73.

[25] Farid NA, Kurihara A, Wrighton SA. Metabolism and disposition of the thienopyridine antiplatelet drugs ticlopidine, clopidogrel, and prasugrel in humans. J Clin Pharmacol 2010; 50: 126-42.

[26] Wallentin L. P2Y(12) inhibitors: differences in properties and mechanisms of action and potential consequences for clinical use. Eur Heart J 2009; 30: 1964-77.

[27] Wiviott SD, Trenk D, Frelinger AL, O'Donoghue M, Neumann FJ, Michelson AD, Angiolillo DJ, Hod H, Montalescot G, Miller DL, Jakubowski JA, Cairns R, Murphy SA, McCabe CH, Antman EM, Braunwald E. PRINCIPLE-TIMI 44 Investigators. Prasugrel compared with high loading and maintenance-dose clopidogrel in patients with planned percutaneous coronary intervention: The Prasugrel in Comparison to Clopidogrel for Inhibition of Platelet Activation and Aggregation-Thrombolysis in Myocardial Infarction 44 trial. Circulation 2007; 116: 2923-32.

[28] Wiviott SD, Braunwald E, McCabe CH, Montalescot G, Ruzyllo W, Gottlieb S, Neumann FJ, Ardissino D, De Servi S, Murphy SA, Riesmeyer J, Weerakkody G, Gibson CM, Antman EM; TRITON-TIMI 38 Investigators. Prasugrel versus clopidogrel in patients with acute coronary syndromes. N Engl J Med 2007; 357: 2001-15.

[29] Cohen M. Oral antiplatelet therapy for acute or chronic management of NSTE ACS: Residual ischemic risk and opportunities for improvement. Cardiovasc Drugs Therap 2009; 23: 489-99.

[30] VAN Giezen JJ, Nilsson L, Berntsson P, Wissing BM, Giordanetto F, Tomlinson W, Greasley PJ. Ticagrelor binds to human P2Y(12) independently from ADP but antagonizes ADP-induced receptor signaling and platelet aggregation. J Thromb Haemost 2009; 7: 1556-65.

[31] Husted S, Emanuelsson H, Heptinstall S, Sandset PM, Wickens M, Peters G. Pharmacodynamics, pharmacokinetics, and safety of the oral reversible P2Y12 antagonist AZD6140 with aspirin in patients with atherosclerosis: a double-blind comparison to clopidogrel with aspirin.Eur Heart J 2006; 27: 1038-47.

[32] Husted S, Harrington RA, Cannon CP, Storey RF, Mitchell P, Emanuelsson H.Bleeding risk with AZD6140, a reversible P2Y12 receptor antagonist, vs. clopidogrel in patients undergoing coronary artery bypass grafting in the DISPERSE2 trial. Int J Clin Pract 2009; 63: 667-70.

[33] Wallentin L, Becker RC, Budaj A, Cannon CP, Emanuelsson H, Held C, Horrow J, Husted S, James S, Katus H, Mahaffey KW, Scirica BM, Skene A, Steg PG,Storey RF, Harrington RA; PLATO Investigators, Freij A, Thorsén M. Ticagrelor versus clopidogrel in patients with acute coronary syndromes. N Engl J Med 2009; 361: 1045-57.

[34] Storey RF, Bliden KP, Patil SB, Karunakaran A, Ecob R, Butler K, Teng R, Wei C, Tantry US, Gurbel PA; ONSET/OFFSET Investigators. Incidence of dyspnea and assessment of cardiac and pulmonary function in patients with stable coronary artery disease receiving ticagrelor, clopidogrel, or placebo in the ONSET/OFFSET study. J Am Coll Cardiol 2010; 56; 185-93.

[35] Michelson AD. P2Y12 antagonism: promises and challenges. Arterioscler Thromb Vasc Biol 2008; 28: 33-38.

[36] Storey RF, Oldroyd KG, Wilcox RG. Open multicentre study of the P2T receptor antagonist AR-C69931MX assessing safety, tolerability and activity in patients with acute coronary syndromes. Thromb Haemost 2001; 85: 401-7.

[37] Bhatt DL, Lincoff AM, Gibson CM, Stone GW, McNulty S, Montalescot G, Kleiman NS, Goodman SG, White HD, Mahaffey KW, Pollack CV Jr, Manoukian SV, Widimsky P, Chew DP, Cura F, Manukov I, Tousek F, Jafar MZ, Arneja J, Skerjanec S, Harrington RA; CHAMPION PLATFORM Investigators.Intravenous platelet blockade with cangrelor during PCI. N Engl J Med 2009; 361: 2330-41.

[38] Harrington RA, Stone GW, McNulty S, White HD, Lincoff AM, Gibson CM, Pollack CV Jr, Montalescot G, Mahaffey KW, Kleiman NS, Goodman SG, Amine M,Angiolillo DJ, Becker RC, Chew DP, French WJ, Leisch F, Parikh KH, Skerjanec S, Bhatt DL. Platelet inhibition with cangrelor in patients undergoing PCI. N Engl J Med 2009; 361: 2318-29.

[39] André P, DeGuzman F, Haberstock-Debic H, Mills S, Pak Y, Inagaki M, Pandey A, Hollenbach S, Phillips DR, Conley PB. Thienopyridines, but not elinogrel, result in off-target effects at the vessel wall that contribute to bleeding. J Pharmacol Exp Ther 2011; 338: 22-30.

[40] Tello-Montoliu A, Tomasello SD, Ueno M, Angiolillo DJ. Antiplatelet therapy: thrombin receptor antagonists. Br J Clin Pharmacol 2011; 72:658-71.

[41] Kahn ML, Zheng YW, Huang W, Bigornia V, Zeng D, Moff S, Farese RV Jr, Tam C, Coughlin SR. A dual thrombin receptor system for platelet activation. Nature 1998; 394: 690–94.

[42] Ji X, Hou M. Novel agents for anti-platelet therapy. J Hematol Oncol 2011; 4: 44.

[43] White HD: Oral anti-platelet therapy for atherothrombotic disease: current evidence and new directions. Am Heart J 2011, 161: 450-61.

[44] Hildemann SK, Bode C: Improving anti-platelet therapy for atherothrombotic disease: preclinical results with SCH 530348, the first oral thrombin receptor antagonist selective for PAR 1. Hamostaseologie 2009, 29: 349-55.

[45] Oestreich J: SCH-530348, a thrombin receptor (PAR-1) antagonist for the prevention and treatment of atherothrombosis. Curr Opin Investig Drugs 2009, 10: 988-96.

[46] Chackalamannil S, Wang Y, Greenlee WJ, Hu Z, Xia Y, Ahn HS, Boykow G, Hsieh Y, Palamanda J, Agans-Fantuzzi J, Kurowski S,Graziano M, Chintala M. Discovery of a novel, orally active himbacine-based thrombin receptor antagonist (SCH 530348) with potent antiplatelet activity. J Med Chem 2008; 51: 3061-4

[47] The TRA·CER Exective and Steering Committees. The Thrombin Receptor Antagonist for Clinical Event Reduction in Acute Coronary Syndrome (TRA·CER) trial: study design and rationale. Am Heart J 2009; 158: 327-34.

[48] Morrow DA, Scirica BM, Fox KA, Berman G, Strony J, Veltri E, Bonaca MP, Fish P, McCabe CH, Braunwald E, TRA 2P-TIMI 50 Investigators. Evaluation of a novel antiplatelet agent for secondary prevention in patients with a history of atherosclerotic disease: design and rationale for the Thrombin-Receptor Antagonist in Secondary Prevention of Atherothrombotic Ischemic Events (TRA 2P)-TIMI 50 trial. Am Heart J 2009; 158: 335-41.

[49] Morrow DA, Braunwald E, Bonaca MP, Ameriso SF, Dalby AJ, Fish MP, Fox KA, Lipka LJ, Liu X, Nicolau JC, Ophuis AJ, Paolasso E, Scirica BM, Spinar J, Theroux P, Wiviott SD, Strony J, Murphy SA; TRA 2P–TIMI 50 Steering Committee and Investigators.Vorapaxar in the secondary prevention of atherothrombotic events. N Engl J Med 2012; 366: 1404-13.

Antiplatelet and Antithrombotic Therapy in Acute Coronary Syndrome in Patients with Chronic Kidney Disease

Mahmut Altındal and Mustafa Arıcı*

Hacettepe University Faculty of Medicine, Department of Nephrology, Ankara, Turkey

Abstract: Chronic kidney disease (CKD) and acute kidney injury (AKI) after acute coronary syndrome (ACS) are strong predictors of morbidity and mortality in patients with ACS. Patients with concomitant kidney and cardiovascular disease constitute a population that is difficult to treat. There are limited data since patients with CKD are usually excluded from cardiovascular studies. Benefits of antiplatelet and antihrombotic therapy must be balanced with risk of adverse events. Kidney function should routinely be evaluated in patients with ACS when such therapies administered. Medications should be used with caution in patients with kidney dysfunction and estimated glomerular filtration rate should be the essential measure used for dosage adjustments. Although additional data are required for evaluation of aspirin's benefit-to-risk ratio in this special population due to inconsistent findings in clinical trials, aspirin is the usual practice and recommended without dose adjustment. Unfractionated heparin, generally do not warrant specific dose adjustment in face of kidney dysfunction. Factor Xa inhibitors, low-molecular-weight heparins and direct thrombin inhibitors except argatroban are predominantly cleared by the kidneys. Reduced doses and frequent monitoring of anticoagulation are indicated when these agents are used in patients with kidney dysfunction. Dose adjustment is usually not required for clopidogrel, prasugrel and ticagrelor in patients with renal impairment. In contrast to abciximab, both eptifibatide and tirofiban are largely eliminated *via* renal excretion thus, careful dose tailoring is warranted among patients with kidney disease.

Keywords: Acute coronary syndrome, antiplatelet therapy, antithrombotic therapy, chronic kidney disease, glomerular filtration rate.

INTRODUCTION

Chronic kidney disease (CKD) is a highly prevalent global health problem. CKD is associated with poor prognosis for patients with acute coronary syndrome

*Corresponding author Mustafa Arici: Hacettepe University Faculty of Medicine Department of Nephrology 06100-Ankara, TURKEY; Tel: +90-312-3051710; Fax: +90-312-3113958; E-mails: marici@hacettepe.edu.tr; aricim@gmail.com

Ertugrul Ercan and Gulfem Ece (Eds.)

(ACS) [1-5]. Although there is increasing information about the effect of acute kidney injury (AKI) on clinical outcomes after ACS, data is scarce in patients with CKD and most data come from retrospective studies [6-9].

CKD is defined as abnormalities of kidney structure or function, present for >3 months, with implications for health [10]. CKD is stratified into five stages based on the level of kidney function (Table 1). Patients with co-existent kidney and cardiovascular disease constitute a difficult-to-treat population. There are limited data since patients with CKD are typically excluded from cardiovascular clinical trials. Although CKD is related with poor outcomes, patients with CKD less frequently receive evidence-based medical therapies than their counterparts with normal kidney function probably due to concerns for adverse effects and potential drug toxicities [11-12]. Uremia, is commonly associated with bleeding tendency but also considered a prothrombotic state [13-15]. The hemostatic defect in uremia is multifactorial and incompletely understood (Fig. 1) [16]. Benefits of antihrombotic therapy must be balanced with perceived risk of bleeding. Kidney function should routinely be assessed in patients with ACS before starting such therapies. In clinical practice, endogenous creatinine is still the substance most widely used to estimate the glomerular filtration rate (GFR) although tubular secretion of creatinine is enhanced in presence of kidney dysfunction which causes overestimation of GFR compared to reference methods [17]. The creatinine clearance is determined from a 24-hour urine collection. Errors in urine collection may underestimate or overestimate creatinine excretion and GFR [18]. Estimated GFR determinations may be performed using Cockroft-Gault, Modification of Diet in Renal Disease (MDRD), or Chronic Kidney Disease Epidemiology Collaboration Research Group (CKD-EPI) equations [10, 19, 20]. CKD-EPI equation is considered more accurate than MDRD, especially when GFR>60 ml/min per 1.73 m^2 [21, 22].

Table 1: GFR categories in CKD

Stage	Terms	GFR (ml/min/1.73 m^2)
G1	Normal or high	≥90
G2	Mildly decreased	60-89
G3a	Mildly to moderately decreased	45-59
G3b	Moderately to severely decreased	30-44
G4	Severely decreased	15-29
G5	Kidney failure	<15

CKD, chronic kidney disease; GFR, glomerular filtration rate.
In the absence of evidence of kidney damage, neither GFR category G1 nor G2 fulfill the criteria for CKD.
Reprinted from the Kidney International with permission [10].

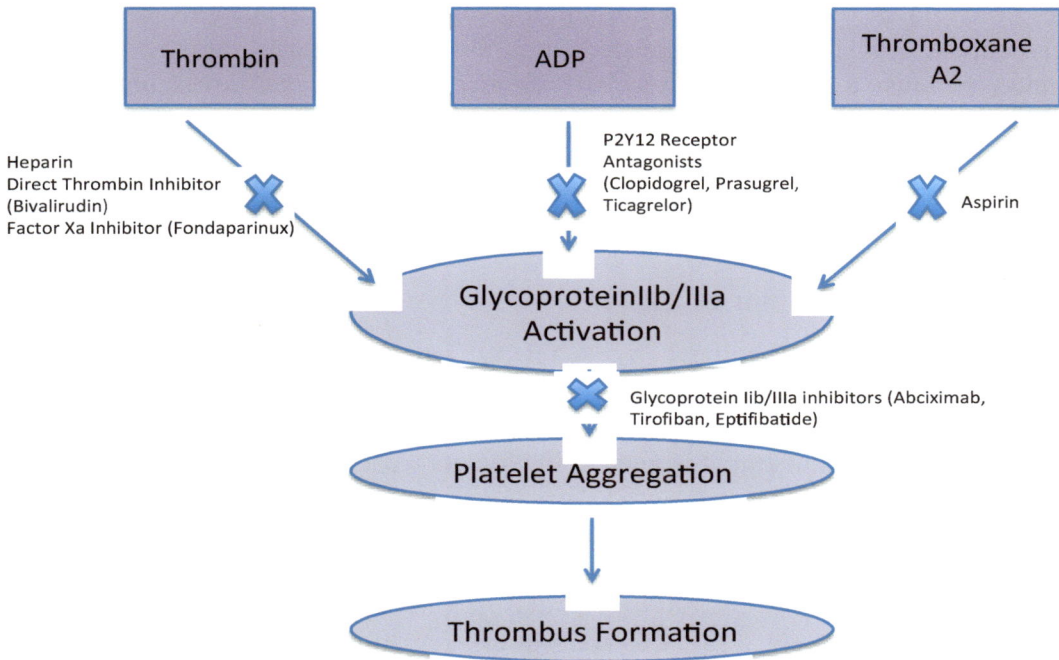

Figure 1: Factors contributing to platelet dysfunction in uremia. (Adopted from Washam *et al.*, Advances in Chronic Kidney Disease with permission [16]).

SUMMARY OF CLINICAL TRIALS AND DRUG ELIMINATION

Aspirin

Most published studies to date with regard to safety and efficiacy of aspirin in patients with CKD gave contradictory findings. The safety of low-dose aspirin was assessed by the first United Kingdom Heart and Renal Protection (UK-HARP-I) study in 448 patients with chronic kidney disease. The study showed that aspirin was associated with a threefold excess of minor bleeds. Although aspirin did not markedly increase the risk for major bleeding, authors concluded that there were too few major bleeds recorded to evaluate safety reliably [23]. The Dialysis Outcomes and Practice Patterns Study (DOPPS) showed that aspirin was associated with a substantial decrease in risk of cerebrovascular accident and did not increase hemorrhagic risk in dialysis patients. In this observational study, low dose aspirin did not decrease cardiovascular morbidity and mortality, even unexpectedly increased cardiac events [24]. In a retrospective study of 595 patients with acute coronary syndrome, aspirin use was an independent predictor of a decreased probability of ST- segment elevation myocardial infarction

(STEMI) [25]. Post- hoc subgroup analysis of the Hypertension Optimal Treatment (HOT) study suggested that low dose aspirin therapy added to antihypertensive treatment prevented significantly more cardiovascular events, and cardiovascular deaths in patients with CKD [26]. The benefit from aspirin therapy increased progressively as eGFR declined. Although risk of major bleeding was greater in the aspirin group than in the placebo group, increased risk of bleeding seemed to be surpassed by the considerable benefit.

Platelet P2y12 Receptor Blockers

Clopidogrel is metabolized by CYP450 enzymes to produce the active metabolite. Following an oral dose of 14C-labeled clopidogrel in humans, close to 50% of total radioactivity was excreted in urine and approximately 46% in feces [27]. No dosage adjustment is needed in patients with renal impairment; however, caution is advised in patients with severe hepatic disease. In a post-hoc analysis of the Clopidogrel for the Reduction of Events During Observation (CREDO) trial population, patients with mild or moderate CKD did not have a significant difference in outcomes (death, myocardial infarction, or stroke) with clopidogrel therapy *versus* placebo [28]. Clopidogrel use increased relative risk of major or minor bleeding, however this increased risk was not different based on renal function. The authors speculated that clopidogrel in mild to moderate CKD patients may not have the same beneficial effect as it does in patients with normal renal function. A post-hoc analysis of the Clopidogrel in Unstable Angina to Prevent Recurrent Events (CURE) trial demonstrated the beneficial effect of adding clopidogrel to standard treatment in non-ST elevation acute coronary syndrome in all three tertiles kidney function although the benefit was not significant in the lowest tertile [29]. The risk of minor bleeding increased in all the three tertiles. The risk of major or life-threatening bleeding moderately increased. These findings suggest that clopidogrel may reduce cardiovascular morbidity and mortality considerably among people with moderate renal impairment and ACS. Park *et al.*, found that, the platelet responsiveness to clopidogrel was decreased in patients with chronic renal failure compared to those with normal renal function, and this decreased platelet responsiveness to clopidogrel was not improved by doubling clopidogrel dosage [30]. Cuisset *et al.*, did not observe any significant effect of CKD on clopidogrel response in patients with ACS, neither for acute response, nor for chronic response with high loading and maintenance clopidogrel doses [31].

Prasugrel, a new thienopyridine derivative, binds irreversibly to platelet P2Y12 receptors and inhibits ADP-induced platelet aggregation [32]. Small *et al.*, investigated the effect of renal impairment on the disposition of prasugrel's active metabolite. There was no difference in pharmacokinetics or pharmacodynamic responses between subjects with moderate renal impairment and healthy subjects, despite lower exposure in subjects with end stage renal disease (ESRD). The platelet aggregation response was comparable in three groups [33].

Ticagrelor, a reversibly binding oral P2Y12 receptor antagonist, yields greater platelet inhibition than clopidogrel [34, 35]. Renal clearance of ticagrelor and its active metabolite is of minor importance [36]. The post-hoc analysis of the Platelet Inhibition and Patient Outcomes (PLATO) trial showed that compared with clopidogrel, ticagrelor significantly reduces ischemic end points and mortality without a significant increase in major bleeding in ACS patients with CKD [37].

Cilastazol

Cilostazol is an oral antiplatelet agent that selectively inhibits phosphodiesterase III [38]. Cilostazol-based triple antiplatelet (aspirin, clopidogrel, and cilostazol) therapy after coronary stenting compared to dual antiplatelet therapy has been associated with a lower rate of adverse cardiovascular outcomes [39-41]. Cilostazol should be used with caution in patients with severe kidney dysfunction (creatinine clearance <25 ml/minute) [42].

Glycoprotein IIb/IIIa Inhibitors

Abciximab is eliminated through the reticuloendothelial system and does not require dose modification in the setting of kidney impairment [43, 44]. Frilling *et al.*, explored the safety and efficacy of abciximab for percutaneous intervention (PCI) in patients with impaired kidney function compared to patients with normal kidney function [45]. Success rates after PCI under abciximab were similar between two groups. Major bleeding was significantly more frequent among patients with impaired kidney function whereas there was no difference in minor bleeding or thrombocytopenia. These data suggested that the effects of abciximab were not entirely independent of kidney function. Pinkau *et al.*, found that, abciximab added to clopidogrel plus aspirin increases the risk of bleeding without benefit in reducing the risk of ischemic complications in patients with kidney disease undergoing PCI [46]. A single center study, performed at the Mayo Clinic demonstrated that, despite the increased risk of bleeding associated with progressive kidney dysfunction in patients undergoing PCI; abciximab did not significantly increase the likelihood of bleeding complications more in patients with CKD than in patients with normal kidney function [47]. Between 39% and 69% of total plasma clearance of **tirofiban**

is *via* kidney [48]. Both the loading dose and the maintenance dose should be reduced by 50% in patients with an estimated creatinine clearance (CrCl) of less than 30 ml/min [49]. A subgroup analysis from PRISM-PLUS (Platelet Receptor Inhibition in Ischemic Syndrome Management in Patients Limited by Unstable Signs and Symptoms) was performed to determine the safety and efficacy of tirofiban in patients with kidney dysfunction [50]. TIMI (Thrombolysis In Myocardial Infarction) major bleeding rates were not significantly higher based on kidney function or the use of tirofiban nevertheless, combined TIMI major and minor bleeding was significantly higher with declining kidney function. In spite of increased bleeding rates, treatment with tirofiban in the presence of kidney dysfunction did not amplify the risk for bleeding further than expected. The authors concluded that among patients with mild-to-moderate kidney disease, tirofiban was well tolerated and effective in reducing ischemic acute coronary syndrome complications. A subgroup analysis of the Do Tirofiban and ReoPro Give Similar Efficacy Outcomes Trial (TARGET) was conducted to determine whether outcome differences exist between tirobifan and abciximab in patients with mild kidney dysfunction [51]. As expected patients with lower creatinine clearance had higher rates of both ischemic and bleeding events. Although tirofiban is cleared from kidneys and abciximab is not, no interaction was observed between the GP IIb/IIIa inhibitor type used and creatinine clearance regarding ischemic or bleeding events. About 40-50% of total body clearance of **eptifibatide** is by the kidneys [52]. Dosage adjustments are necessary in patients with creatinine clearances less than 50 ml/min/1.73m^2. An analysis of (PROTECT-TIMI-30) trial supported that among non ST-segment elevation acute coronary syndrome, percutaneous intervention (NSTE-ACS PCI) patients treated with eptifibatide, use of creatinine CrCl or GFR may be preferable to serum creatinine to adjust eptifibatide dosing [53]. Administration of full dose eptifibatide to patients with reduced CrCl, was associated with a greater incidence of bleeding events. Results of a prospective observational analysis of patients from the CRUSADE (Can Rapid Risk Stratification of Unstable Angina Patients Suppress Adverse Outcomes With Early Implementation of the American College of Cardiology/American Heart Association Guidelines) National Quality Improvement Initiative Registry proved that excess doses of GPIIb/IIIa inhibitors were administered to patients with NSTE-ACS in community [54]. The risk of major bleeding due to dosing errors was increased especially in vulnerable subgroups including women, elderly and patients with kidney dysfunction.

Indirect Thrombin Inhibitors

At low doses, **unfractionated heparin** (UFH) is cleared primarily by the cellular or saturable mechanisms, *via* binding to macrophages and endothelial cells. At greater doses, after cellular binding becomes saturated; the kidney or nonsaturable mechanism becomes more eminent [55-57]. UFH reduces mortality and cardiac reinfarction within 30 days in patients with ACS, however data concerning its safety and effectiveness was limited in patients with ACS with CKD [58].

Low molecular weight heparins (LMWHs) are eliminated primarily by kidneys [58]. Becker *et al.*, showed that severe kidney dysfunction (creatinine clearance < 40 ml/min) significantly affects enoxaparin's anti-Xa pharmacokinetics and pharmacodynamics, which leads to higher anti-Xa activity and increased incidence of major bleeding in patients with ACS [59]. In a substudy of the EXTRACT-TIMI 25 (Enoxaparin and Thrombolysis Reperfusion for Acute Myocardial Infarction Treatment) trial, there were increment of the risk of major or minor bleeding by approximately 50% with each successive 30-ml/min diminution of CrCl [60]. There are limited clinical data on the safety of dalteparin and tinzaparin in patients with kidney dysfunction. A retrospective subgroup analyses was performed using the combined data from the Thrombolysis in Myocardial Infarction (TIMI) 11B and Efficacy Safety Subcutaenous Enoxaparin in Non-Q-wave Coronary Events (ESSENCE) trials. There were higher rates of major and any bleeding events in patients with NSTE-ACS and severe kidney dysfunction than in patients with NSTE-ACS without kidney disease in both groups treated with UFH or enoxaparin [61]. Anti-Xa monitoring (peak level 4-6 hours after SC injection) is recommended in patients with severe kidney disease (CrCl <30 ml/min) who are receiving LMWH at therapeutic doses.

Direct Thrombin Inhibitors

Plasma clearance of **bivalirudin** decreases with impaired renal function [62]. In a subanalysis of the The Randomized Evaluation in PCI Linking Angiomax to Reduced Clinical Events (REPLACE)-2 trial [63], Chew *et al.*, compared bivalirudin to heparin and glycoprotein IIb/IIIa inhibition with regard to ischemic and bleeding events among patients with renal impairment undergoing percutaneous coronary intervention. Bivalirudin suppressed ischemic events similar to heparin and glycoprotein IIb/IIIa inhibition irrespective of renal impairment. Bleeding events were fewer regardlesss of kidney function [64].

Argatroban compared with heparin, enhances reperfusion with tissue plasminogen activator (TPA) in patients with AMI, particularly in those patients with delayed presentation [65-66]. Although no dosage adjustment of argatroban is required in patients with renal impairment due to its minimal excretion by kidneys, close monitoring with aPTT is recommended in patients with severe kidney disease [67-68].

Factor Xa Inhibitors

Fondaparinux is almost completely excreted by the kidneys [69]. Fondaparinux is contraindicated in severe kidney disease [70]. Fox *et al.*, conducted a subgroup analysis of the OASIS-5 (Fifth Organization to Assess Strategies in Acute Coronary Syndrome) to compare the efficacy and safety of fondaparinux with enoxaparin when administered for non-ST-segment elevation ACS over the spectrum of kidney dysfunction [71]. The absolute differences in composite end point and bleeding in favor of fondaparinux were most remarkable in patients with a GFR less than 58 ml/min per 1.73 m^2.

CLINICAL APPROACH AND PRACTICE GUIDELINES

American College of Cardiology Foundation/American Heart Association (ACCF/AHA) guidelines suggest that all patients with cardiovascular disease should be screened for kidney disease by estimating GFR, testing for microalbuminuria, and measuring the albumin-to-creatinine ratio. These guidelines propose that GFR less than 60 mL/min/1.73m^2 and albumin-to-creatinine ratio greater than 30 mg of albumin per 1 g of creatinine should be regarded as abnormal [72]. The diagnosis of ACS in presence of kidney dysfunction may be problematic in absence of apparent ECG findings. Serum cardiac troponin levels may be increased in patients with reduced kidney function without active cardiac ischemia [73]. Cardiac TnI is elevated less frequently than cardiac TnT in setting of kidney dysfunction. Although TnI and TnT are comparable in diagnosis and prognosis of acute coronary syndromes, TnI may be more spesific in case of kidney dysfuntion [74-76]. Patients with ACS and CKD either don't receive evidence-based therapies due to concerns for bleeding or overdosed with antithrombotics when kidney function was not taken into account. Medications should be used with extreme caution in patients with kidney dysfunction and the estimated glomerular filtration rate (eGFR) should be the primary measure for dose adjustments [72, 77].

Unstable Angina/Non-ST-Segment Elevation Myocardial Infarction

Table 2 summarizes the most recent European Society of Cardiology (ESC) guidelines for patients with CKD and non-ST-segment elevation-ACS. Table **3** shows the recommendations for antithrombotic agents. Available data is meager to draw a definitive algorithm for management of this special group of patients. An opinion-based algorithm for unstable angina/non-ST-segment elevation myocardial infarction (UA/NSTEMI) based on ACCF/AHA and ESC guidelines is presented below (Fig. **2**). If invasive management strategy is selected, preventive measures should be taken to minimize risk of contrast-induced nephropathy (Table **2**).

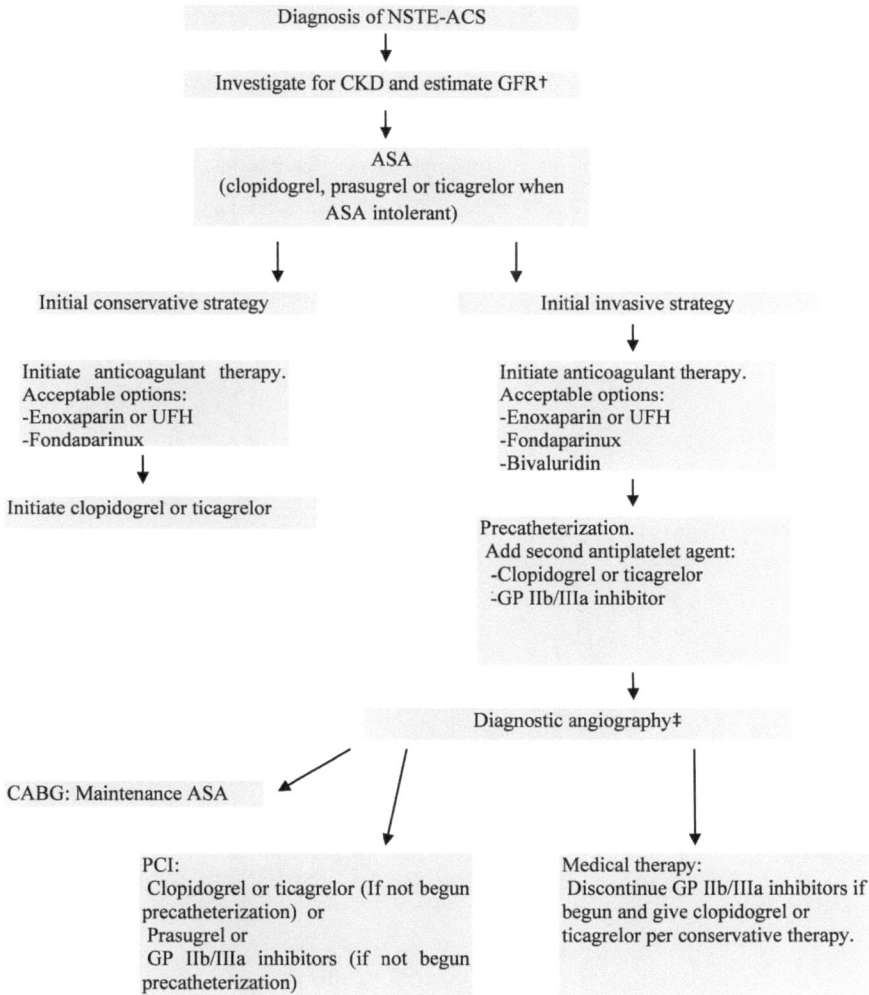

Figure 2: Algorithm for management of NSTE-ACS in patients with chronic kidney disease*
†See text.
*See Tables **1** to **4** for dosing issues in CKD.
‡ See Table **2**.
ASA = aspirin; CABG = coronary artery bypass graft; GP = glycoprotein; PCI = percutaneous coronary intervention; UA/NSTEMI = unstable angina/ ST-elevation myocardial infarction; UFH = unfractionated heparin.
Adopted from Anderson *et al.,* /JACC [72].

ST-Segment Elevation Myocardial Infarction

There are no clear guidelines for management ST-segment elevation myocardial infarction (STEMI) in patients with kidney dysfunction. In patients presenting with STEMI and reduced kidney function, some of the antithrombotic drugs may be changed or proper dose adjustment is required [78] (Table **4**).

Table 2: ESC Guidelines for the management of acute coronary syndromes in patients presenting without persistent ST-segment elevation: Recommendations for patients with CKD.

Recommendations	Class [a]	Level [b]
Kidney function should be assessed by CrCl or eGFR in patients with NSTE-ACS with special attention to elderly people, woman, patients with low body weight, as near normal serum creatinine levels may be associated with lower than expected CrCl and eGFR levels.	I	C
Patients with NSTE-ACS and CKD should receive the same first-line antithrombotic treatment as patients devoid of CKD, with appropriate dose adjustments according to severity of renal function.	I	B
Depending degree of renal dysfunction, dose adjustment or switch to UFH with fondaparinux, enoxaparin, bivalirudin, as well as dose adjustment with small molecule GP IIb/IIIa receptor inhibitors are indicated.	I	B
UFH infusion adjusted to aPTT is recommended when CrCl is<30 ml/min or eGFR is <30 ml/min/1.73 m^2 with most anticoagulants (fondaparinux <20 ml/min).	I	C
In patients with NSTE-ACS and CKD considered for invasive strategy, hydration and low- or iso-osmolar contrast medium at low volume (<4 mL/kg) are recommended.	I	B
CABG or PCI is recommended in patients with CKD amenable to revascularization after careful assessment of the risk-benefit ratio in relation to the severity of renal dysfunction.	I	B

[a]Class of recommendation.
[b]Level of evidence.
aPTT = activated partial thromboplastin time; CABG = coronary artery bypass graft; CKD = chronic kidney disease; CrCl = creatinine clearance; eGFR = estimated glomerular filtration rate; GP = glycoprotein; NSTE-ACS = non-ST-elevation acute coronary syndrome; PCI = percutaneous coronary intervention; UFH = unfractionated heparin.
Reprinted from Hamm *et al.*,/ Eur Heart J [77].

Table 3: ESC Guidelines for the management of acute coronary syndromes in patients presenting without persistent ST-segment elevation: Recommendations for use of antithrombotic drugs in CKD.

Drug	Recommendations
Clopidogrel	No information in patients with renal dysfunction.
Prasugrel	No dose adjustment necessary, including in patients with end-stage disease.
Ticagrelor	No dose reduction required; no information in dialysis patients.
Enoxaparin	Dose reduction to 1 mg/kg once daily in the case of severe renal failure (CrCl <30 mL/min). Consider monitoring of anti-Xa activity.
Fondaparinux	Contraindicated in severe renal failure (CrCl <20 mL/min). Drug of choice in patients with moderately reduced renal function (CrCl 30–60 mL/min).
Bivalirudin	Patients with moderate renal impairment (30-59 mL/min) should receive an infusion of 1.75 mg/kg/h. If the creatinine clearance is <30 mL/min, reduction of the infusion rate to 1 mg/kg/h should be considered. No reduction in the bolus dose is needed. If a patient is on haemodialysis, the infusion rate should be reduced to 0.25 mg/kg/h.
Abciximab	No specific recommendations for the use of abciximab, or for dose adjustment in the case of renal failure. Careful evaluation of haemorrhagic risk is needed before using the drug in the case of renal failure.
Eptibifatide	The infusion dose should be reduced to 1 µg/kg/min in patients with CrCl <50 mL/min. The dose of the bolus remains unchanged at 180 µg/kg. Eptifibatide is contraindicated in patients with CrCl <30 mL/min.
Tirobifan	Dose adaptation is required in patients with renal failure; 50% of the bolus dose and infusion if CrCl is <30 mL/min.

Recommendations for the use of drugs listed in this table may vary depending on the exact labelling of each drug in the country where it is used.
CrCl= Creatinine clearance.
Reprinted from Hamm *et al*./ Eur Heart J [77].

Table 4: ESC Guidelines for the management of acute myocardial infarction in patients presenting with ST-segment elevation: Initial dosing of antithrombotic agents in patients with CKD (estimated creatinine clearance <60 mL/min)

Drug	Recommendations
Aspirin	No dose adjustment.
Clopidogrel	No dose adjustment.
Prasugrel	No dose adjustment. No experience with end-stage renal disease/dialysis.

Ticagrelor	No dose adjustment. No experience with end-stage renal disease/dialysis.
Enoxaparin	No adjustment of bolus dose. Following thrombolysis, in patients with creatinine clearance <30 mL/min, the s.c. doses are given once every 24 h.
Unfractinated heparin	No adjustment of bolus dose.
Fondaparinux	No dose adjustment. No experience in patients with end-stage renal disease or dialysis patients.
Bivaluridin	• In patients with moderate renal insufficiency (GFR 30-59 mL/min) a lower initial infusion rate of 1.4 mg/kg/h should be given. The bolus dose should not be changed. • In patients with severe renal insufficiency (GFR <30 mL/min) and in dialysis-dependent patients bivalirudin is contraindicated.
Abciximab	No specific recommendation. Careful consideration of bleeding risk.
Eptibifatide	• In patients with moderate renal insufficiency (GFR ≥30 to <50 mL/min), an i.v. bolus of 180 μg should be administered followed by a continuous infusion dose of 1.0 μg/kg/min for the duration of therapy. • In patients with severe renal insufficiency (GFR <30 mL/min) eptifibatide is contraindicated.
Tirobifan	In patients with severe renal insufficiency (GFR <30 mL/min) the infusion dose should be reduced to 50%.

GFR=Glomerular filtration rate.
Reprinted from Steg *et al.*/European Heart Journal [78].

NOVEL DRUGS

Apixaban is an orally active, direct-acting, factor Xa inhibitor. Its use should be avoided in patients with creatinine clearance CrCl <15 ml/min/1.73m^2 and it should be used with caution in patients with severe kidney dysfunction (CrCl 15-29 ml/min/1.73m^2) [79]. In patients with atrial fibrillation, apixaban has been found to be superior to warfarin in preventing stroke or systemic embolism [80]. It decreases the incidence of venous thromboembolism in patients undergoing orthopedic surgery [81]. Apixaban failed to reduce ischemic events when added to antiplatelet therapy in high-risk patients after an acute coronary syndrome and it increased the number of major bleeding events [82].

Rivaroxaban is an orally available direct factor Xa inhibitor. Rivaroxaban use is not advocated in patients with CrCl <15 ml/min [83]. Rivaroxaban has been found to be non-inferior to warfarin for the prevention of stroke or systemic embolism and in prevention of stroke and systemic embolism in patients with nonvalvular atrial fibrillation [84]. Rivaroxaban is effective both in prevention and treatment of venous thromboembolism [85, 86]. In patients with a recent acute coronary syndrome, ATLAS ACS-TIMI 51 (The Anti-Xa Therapy to Lower cardiovascular events in addition to Aspirin with or without thienopyridine therapy in Subjects with Acute Coronary Syndrome–Thrombolysis In Myocardial Infarction 51) phase III trial showed that rivaroxaban reduced the risk of the composite end point of death from cardiovascular causes, myocardial infarction, or stroke at the expense of increased the risk of major bleeding and intracranial hemorrhage [87].

Dabigatran is an oral direct thrombin inhibitor. Exposure to dabigatran is increased by kidney dysfunction due to its predominantly (up to 80%) renal elimination [88]. There is insufficient data regarding its use in patients with severe kidney disease (CrCl <15 ml/min or on dialysis) [89]. Dabigatran has been shown to be non-inferior to enoxaparin in prevention of VTE following orthopedic surgery [90, 91]. For the treatment of acute venous thromboembolism, dabigatran has found to have a similar efficacy and safety profile with warfarin [92]. In patients with atrial fibrillation, dabigatran given at at a dose of 150 mg, was associated with lower rates of stroke and systemic embolism compared to warfarin but similar rates of major hemorrhage [93]. The Randomised Dabigatran Etexilate Dose Finding Study In Patients With Acute Coronary Syndromes Post Index Event With Additional Risk Factors For Cardiovascular Complications Also Receiving Aspirin And Clopidogrel (RE-DEEM) study suggested that dabigatran, in addition to dual antiplatelet therapy, was associated with a dose-dependent increase in bleeding events and significantly reduced coagulation activity in patients with a recent myocardial infarction [94]. In a post-hoc analysis of The Randomized Evaluation of Long-term Anticoagulant Therapy (RE-LY) trial, there was a nonsignificant increase in MI with dabigatran compared with warfarin in patients with atrial fibrillation [95]. A meta-analysis of seven randomized trials showed that dabigatran was associated with a significantly increased risk of myocardial infarction or acute coronary syndrome when compared with warfarin, enoxaparin or placebo [96].

Vorapaxar (SCH 530348) is an orally active, reversible, and selective inhibitor of the protease-activated receptor-1 thrombin receptor (PAR 1). It is inactivated *via* the CYP3A4 system, the kidney metabolism is negligible [97]. In patients with acute coronary syndromes, the addition of vorapaxar to standard therapy did not significantly reduce the ischemic events and the primary composite end point but significantly increased the risk of major bleeding [98].

Atopaxar is an orally available PAR 1 antagonist that interferes with platelet signaling. It is also metabolized by the CYP3A4 system [97]. The Lessons From Antagonizing the Cellular Effects of Thrombin-Acute Coronary Syndromes (LANCELOT-ACS) trial suggested that in patients after ACS, atopaxar significantly reduced early ischemia on Holter monitoring without a significant increase in major or minor bleeding [99]. Larger trials are required evaluate the efficacy and safety of atopaxar.The characteristics of new oral anticoagulants are summarized in Table **5** [100]. Novel oral anticoagulants may prevent or reduce future cardiovascular events but the bleeding risk should be carefully evaluated.

Table 5: Novel oral anticoagulants recently evaluated in ACS

Drug	Class	Half life	Excretion	Tolerability	Interactions
Apixaban	Direct factor Xa inhibitor	8-14 h	25% Urine 25% Feces Liver	No unexpected safety concerns	Strong CYP enzyme inducers and inhibitors
Rivaroxaban	Direct factor Xa inhibitor	7-9 h	Urine, feces, biliary system	No unexpected safety concerns	Potent CYP3A4 inducers, P-gp/CYP3A4 inhibitors
Darexaban	Direct factor Xa inhibitor	14-18 h	50% Urine 50% Feces	No unexpected safety concerns	No known drug–drug interactions
Dabigatran	Direct thrombin inhibitor	12-18 h	80% Urine	Risk of MI	P-gp inhibitors and inducers
Vorapaxar	PAR 1 antagonist	126-269 h	Gastrointestinal and biliary tracts	Excess of intracranial hemorrhage in patients with PMH of stroke	CYP3A4 inducers and inhibitors
Atoxapar	PAR 1 antagonist	22–26 h	Gastrointestinal metabolism	Liver toxicity, QT prolongation	CYP3A4 inducers and inhibitors

Adopted from Costopoulos *et al.*/International Journal of Cardiology with permission [100].

ACKNOWLEDGEMENTS

Declared none.

CONFLICT OF INTEREST

The authors confirm that this chapter contents have no conflict of interest.

REFERENCES

[1]   Reddan DN, Szczech L, Bhapkar MV, *et al.* Renal function, concomitant medication use and outcomes following acute coronary syndromes. Nephrol Dial Transplant 2005; 20: 2105-12.

[2]   Wright RS, Reeder GS, Herzog CA, *et al.* Acute myocardial infarction and renal dysfunction: a high-risk combination. Ann Intern Med 2002; 137: 563.

[3]   Santopinto JJ, Fox KA, Goldberg RJ, *et al.* Creatinine clearance and adverse hospital outcomes in patients with acute coronary syndromes: Findings from the global registry of acute coronary events (GRACE). Heart 2003; 89: 1003-8.

[4]   Gibson CM, Dumaine RL, Gelfand EV, *et al.* Association of glomerular filtration rate on presentation with subsequent mortality in non-STsegment elevation acute coronary syndrome: Observations in 13,307 patients in five TIMI trials. Eur Heart J 2004; 25: 1998-2005.

[5]   Mielniczuk LM, Pfeffer MA, Lewis EF, *et al.* Estimated glomerular filtration rate, inflammation, and cardiovascular events after an acute coronary syndrome. Am Heart J 2008; 155: 725-31.

[6]   Goldberg A, Hammerman H, Petcherski S, *et al.* Inhospital and 1-year mortality of patients who develop worsening renal function following acute ST-elevation myocardial infarction. Am Heart J 2005; 150: 330-337.

[7]   Newsome BB, Warnock DG, McClellan WM, *et al.* Long-term risk of mortality and end-stage renal disease among the elderly after small increases in serum creatinine level during hospitalization for acute myocardial infarction. Arch Intern Med 2008; 168: 609-16.

[8]   Parikh CR, Coca SG, Wang Y, *et al.* Long-term prognosis of acute kidney injury after acute myocardial infarction. Arch Intern Med 2008; 168: 987-995.

[9]   Rodrigues FB, Bruetto RG, Torres US, *et al.* Effect of kidney disease on acute coronary syndrome. Clin J Am Soc Nephrol 2010; 5(8): 1530-6.

[10]   KDIGO. Kidney International Supplements 2013; 3: 19-62

[11]   Yan AT, Yan RT, Tan M, *et al.* Treatment and one-year outcome of patients with renal dysfunction across the broad spectrum of acute coronary syndromes. Can J Cardiol 2006; 22(2): 115-20.

[12]   Fox CS, Muntner P, Chen AY, *et al.* Use of evidence-based therapies in short-term outcomes of ST-segment elevation myocardial infarction and non-ST-segment elevation myocardial infarction in patients with chronic kidney disease: a report from the National Cardiovascular Data Acute Coronary Treatment and Intervention Outcomes Network registry. Circulation 2010; 121: 357-65.

[13]   Wattanakit K, Kushman M, Stehman-Breen C, *et al.* Chronic kidney disease increases risk for venous thromboembolism. J Am Soc Nephrol 2008; 19: 135-40.

[14]   Mezzano D, Tagle R, Panes O, *et al.* Hemostatic disorder of uremia: the platelet defect, main determinant of the prolonged bleeding time, is correlated with indices of activation of coagulation and fibrinolysis. Thromb Haemost 1996; 76: 312-21.

[15]   Castillo R, Lozano T, Escolar G, *et al.* Defective platelet adhesion on vessel subendothelium in uremic patients. Blood 1986; 68: 337-42.

[16]   Washam JB, Adams G. Risks and benefits of antiplatelet therapy in uremic patients. Adv Chronic Kidney Dis 2008; 15: 370-7.

[17]   Shemesh O, Golbetz H, Kriss J *et al.* Limitations of creatinine as a filtration marker in glomerulopathic patients. Kidney Int 1985; 28: 830.

[18]   Rose BD, Post TW. Clinical Physiology of Acid-Base and Electrolyte Disorders, 5th ed. New York: McGraw-Hill 2001; pp. 50-57.

[19]   Levy AS, Lewis JB, Bosch JP, *et al.* A more accurate method to estimate glomerular filtration rate from serum creatinine: A new prediction equation. Modification of Diet in Renal Disease Study Group. Ann Internal Med 1999; 130: 461-70.

[20]   Cockcroft DW, Gault MH. Prediction of creatinine clearance from serum creatinine. Nephron 1976; 16: 31-41.

[21]   Stevens LA, Coresh J, Feldman HI, *et al*. Evaluation of the modification of diet in renal disease study equation in a large diverse population. J Am Soc Nephrol 2007; 18: 2749-57.

[22]   Levey AS, Stevens LA, Schmid CH, *et al*. A new equation to estimate glomerular filtration rate. Ann Intern Med 2009; 150: 604-12.

[23]   Baigent C, Landray M, Leaper C, *et al*. First United Kingdom Heart and Renal Protection (UK-HARP-I) study: biochemical efficacy and safety of simvastatin and safety of low-dose aspirin in chronic kidney disease. Am J Kidney Dis 2005; 45: 473.

[24]   Ethier J, Bragg-Gresham JL, Piera L, *et al*. Aspirin prescription and outcomes in hemodialysis patients: the Dialysis Outcomes and Practice Patterns Study (DOPPS). Am J Kidney Dis 2007; 50: 602.

[25]   Sciahbasi A, Arcieri R, Quarto M, *et al*. Impact of chronic aspirin and statin therapy on presentation of patients with acute myocardial infarction and impaired renal function. Prev Cardiol 2010; 13: 18-22.

[26]   Jardine MJ, Ninomiya T, Perkovic V, *et al*. Aspirin is beneficial in hypertensive patients with chronic kidney disease: a post-hoc subgroup analysis of a randomized controlled trial. J Am Coll Cardiol 2010; 56: 95.

[27]   Bristol-Myers Squibb/Sanofi Pharmaceuticals Partnership: Clopidogrel (Plavix) prescribing information. Bridgewater, NJ 08807, December 2011. Available from http: //packageinserts.bms.com/pi/pi_plavix.pdf.

[28]   Best PJ, Steinhubl SR, Berger PB, *et al*. The efficacy and safety of short- and long-term dual antiplatelet therapy in patients with mild or moderate chronic kidney disease: results from the Clopidogrel for the Reduction of Events During Observation (CREDO) trial. Am Heart J 2008; 155: 687-93.

[29]   Keltai M, Tonelli M, Mann JF, *et al*: CURE Trial Investigators. Renal function and outcomes in acute coronary syndrome: impact of clopidogrel. Eur J Cardiovasc Prev Rehabil 2007 Apr; 14(2): 312-8.

[30]   Park SH, Kim W, Park CS, *et al*. A comparison of clopidogrel responsiveness in patients with *versus* without chronic renal failure. Am J Cardiol 2009; 104: 1292-5.

[31]   Cuisset T, Frere C, Moro PJ, *et al*. Lack of effect of chronic kidney disease on clopidogrel response with high loading and maintenance doses of clopidogrel after acute coronary syndrome. Thromb Res. 2010 ; 126(5): e400-2.

[32]   Jakubowski JA, Winters KJ, Naganuma H, *et al*. Prasugrel: a novel thienopyridine antiplatelet agent. A review of preclinical and clinical studies and the mechanistic basis for its distinct antiplatelet profile. Cardiovascular Drug Review, 2007; 25, 357-74.

[33]   Small DS, Wrishko RE, Ernest CS, *et al*. Prasugrel pharmacokinetics and pharmacodynamics in subjects with moderate renal impairment and end-stage renal disease. J Clin Pharm Ther 2009; 34: 585-94.

[34]   Gurbel PA, Bliden KP, Butler K, Antonino MJ, *et al*. Response to ticagrelor in clopidogrel nonresponders and responders and effect of switching therapies: the RESPOND Study. Circulation. 2010; 121: 1188-99.

[35]   Wallentin L, Becker RC, Budaj A, *et al*. Ticagrelor *versus* clopidogrel in patients with acute coronary syndromes. N Engl J Med 2009; 361: 1045-57.

[36]   Husted S, van Giezen JJ. Ticagrelor: The first reversibly binding oral $P2Y_{12}$ receptor antagonist. Cardiovasc Ther 2009; 27: 259-74.

[37]   James S, Budaj A, Aylward P, *et al*. Ticagrelor *versus* clopidogrel in acute coronary syndromes in relation to renal function: results from the Platelet Inhibition and Patient Outcomes (PLATO) trial. Circulation 2010; 122: 1056-67.

[38]   Kambayashi J, Liu Y, Sun B, *et al*. Cilostazol as a unique antithrombotic agent. Curr Pharm Des 2003; 9: 2289-302.

[39]   Lee SW, Park SW, Hong MK, *et al*. Triple *versus* dual antiplatelet therapy after coronary stenting: impact on stent thrombosis. J Am Coll Cardiol 2005; 46: 1833.

[40]   Han Y, Li Y, Wang S, *et al*. Cilostazol in addition to aspirin and clopidogrel improves long-term outcomes after percutaneous coronary intervention in patients with acute coronary syndromes: a randomized, controlled study. Am Heart J 2009; 157: 733.

[41]   Chen KY, Rha SW, Li YJ, *et al*. Triple *versus* dual antiplatelet therapy in patients with acute ST-segment elevation myocardial infarction undergoing primary percutaneous coronary intervention. Circulation 2009; 119: 3207.
[42]   *Otsuka America Pharmaceuticals Incorporation: Pletal prescribing information*. Rockville, MD 20850, May 2007. Available from *http: //*www.otsuka-us.com/Products/Documents/Pletal.
[43]   Anderson JR, and Riding D. Glycoprotein IIb/IIIa Inhibitors in Patients With Renal Insufficiency Undergoing Percutaneous Coronary Intervention. Cardiology in Review 2008; 16: 213-218.
[44]   Eli Lilly and Company: Reopro (Abciximab) for Intravenous Administration prescribing information.Indianapolis, IN 46285, No Indianapolis, November 2005. Available from http: //www.janssenbiotech.com/assets/reopro.pdf.
[45]   Frilling B, Zahn B, Mark B, *et al*. Comparison of efficacy and complication rates after percutaneous coronary interventions in patients with and without renal insufficiency treated with abciximab. Am J Cardiol. 2002; 89: 450- 52.
[46]   Pinkau T, Ndrepepa G, Kastrati A, *et al*. Glycoprotein IIb/IIIa receptor inhibition with abciximab during percutaneous coronary interventions increases the risk of bleeding in patients with impaired renal function. Cardiology 2008; 111: 247-53.
[47]   Best PJ, Lennon R, Gersh BJ, *et al*. Safety of abciximab in patients with chronic renal insufficiency who are undergoing percutaneous coronary interventions. Am Heart J. 2003; 146: 345-50.
[48]   Medicure Pharma Incorporation: Aggrastat prescribing information. Summerset, NJ 08873 USA, May 2012. Available from http//: www.medicure.com/aggrastat/aggrastat.html.
[49]   Bhatt DL, Topol EJ. Current role of platelet glycoprotein IIb/IIIa inhibitors in acute coronary syndromes. JAMA 2000; 284: 1549-1558.
[50]   Januzzi JL, Snapinn SM, DiBattiste PM, *et al*. Benefits and safety of tirofiban among acute coronary syndrome patients with mild to moderate renal insufficiency. Circulation 2002; 105: 2361-2366.
[51]   Berger PB, Best PJ, Topol EJ, *et al*. The relation of renal function to ischemic and bleeding outcomes with 2 different glycoprotein IIb/IIIa inhibitors: the do tirofiban and ReoPro give similar efficacy outcome (TARGET) trial. Am Heart J 2005; 149: 869-75.
[52]   Alton KB, Kosoglou T, Baker S, *et al*. Disposition of 14C-eptifibatide after intravenous administration to healthy men. Clin Ther 1998; 20: 307-323.
[53]   Kirtane AJ, Piazza G, Murphy SA, *et al*. Correlates of bleeding events among moderate-to high risk patients undergoing percutaneous coronary intervention and treated with eptifibatide: observations from the PROTECT-TIMI-30 Trial. J Am Coll Cardiol 2006; 47: 2374-79.
[54]   Alexander KP, Chen AY, Roe MT, *et al*. Excess dosing of antiplatelet and antithrombin agents in the treatment of non-ST-segment elevation acute coronary syndromes. JAMA. 2005; 294: 3108-16.
[55]   Follea G, Laville M, Pozet N, *et al*. Pharmacokinetic studies of standard heparin and low molecular weight heparin in patients with chronic renal failure. Haemostasis 1986; 16: 147-51.
[56]   Boneu B, Caanobe C, Cadroy Y, *et al*: Pharmacokinetic studies of standard unfractionated heparin, and low molecular weight heparins in the rabbit. Semin Thromb Haemost 1988; 14: 18-27.
[57]   Maison, AG, Charest AF and Geerts WH. Anticoagulant Use in Patients with Chronic Renal Impairment. Am J Cardiovasc Drugs 2005; 5 (5): 291-305.
[58]   Gilchrist IC, Berkowitz SD, Thompson TD, *et al*. Heparin dosing and outcome in acute coronary syndromes: the GUSTO-IIb experience. Global Use of Strategies to Open Occluded Coronary Arteries. Am Heart J 2002; 144: 73-80.
[59]   Becker RC, Spencer FA, Gibson M, *et al*. Influence of patient characteristics and renal function on factor Xa inhibition pharmacokinetics and pharmacodynamics after enoxaparin administration in non-ST-segment elevation acute coronary syndromes. Am Heart J 2002; 143: 753-9.
[60]   Fox KA, Antman EM, Montalescot G, *et al*. The impact of renal dysfunction on outcomes in the EXTRACT-TIMI 25 trial. J Am Coll Cardiol 2007; 49: 2249 -55.
[61]   Spinler SA, Inverso SM, Cohen M *et al*. Safety and efficacy of unfractionated heparin *versus* enoxaparin in patients who are obese and patients with severe renal impairment: analysis from the ESSENCE and TIMI 11B studies. Am Heart J 2003; 146: 33-41.
[62]   Robson R, White H, Aylward P, Frampton C. Bivalirudin pharmacokinetics and pharmacodynamics: effect of renal function, dose, and gender. Clin Pharmacol Ther. 2002; 71(6): 433-9.
[63]   Lincoff A.M., Bittl J.A., Harrington R.A. *et al*. Bivalirudin and provisional glycoprotein IIb/IIIa blockade compared with heparin and planned glycoprotein IIb/IIIa blockade during percutaneous coronary intervention: REPLACE-2 randomized trial. JAMA 2003; 289: 853-863.

[64] Chew DP, Lincoff AM, Gurm H *et al*. Bivalirudin *versus* heparin and glycoprotein IIb/IIIa inhibition among patients with renal impairment undergoing percutaneous coronary intervention (a subanalysis of the REPLACE-2 trial).Am J Cardiol. 2005; 95(5): 581-5.

[65] Clarke RJ, Mayo G, FitzGerald GA, *et al*. Combined administration of aspirin and a specific thrombin inhibitor in man. Circulation 1991; 83: 1510.

[66] Jang IK, Brown DF, Giugliano RP, *et al*. A multicenter, randomized study of argatroban *versus* heparin as adjunct to tissue plasminogen activator (TPA) in acute myocardial infarction: myocardial infarction with novastan and TPA (MINT) study. J Am Coll Cardiol 1999; 33: 1879.

[67] Swan SK, Hursting MJ. The pharmacokinetics and pharmacodynamics of argatroban: effects of age, gender, and hepatic or renal dysfunction. Pharmacotherapy 2000; 20: 318-29.

[68] GlaxoSmithKline: Argatroban prescribing information. Research Triangle Park, NC: 27709, April 2012. Available from http: //www.gsksource.com.

[69] Bauer KA New. Pentasaccharides for Prophylaxis of Deep Vein Thrombosis: Pharmacology. Chest 2003; 124; 364S-70S.

[70] GlaxoSmithKline: Arixtra (fondaparinux sodium [injection]) prescribing information. Research Triangle Park, NC 27709, 2011 February. Available from https: //www.gsksource.com.

[71] Fox KA, Bassand JP, Mehta SR, *et al*. Influence of renal function on the efficacy and safety of fondaparinux relative to enoxaparin in non ST-segment elevation acute coronary syndromes. Ann Intern Med 2007; 147: 304-10.

[72] Anderson JL, Adams CD, Antman EM *et al*. 2012 ACCF/AHA focused update incorporated into the ACCF/AHA 2007 guidelines for the management of patients with unstable angina/non-ST-elevation myocardial infarction: a report of the American College of Cardiology Foundation/American Heart Association Task Force on Practice Guidelinesl. J Am Coll Cardiol. 2013; 61(23): e179-347.

[73] Freda BJ, Tang WH, Van Lente F, Peacock WF, Francis GS. Cardiac troponins in renal insufficiency: review and clinical implications. J Am Coll Cardiol. 2002; 40: 2065-71.

[74] Martin GS, Becker BN, Schulman G. Cardiac troponin-I accurately predicts myocardial injury in renal failure. Nephrol Dial Transplant 1998; 13: 1709-12.

[75] Apple FS, Sharkey SW, Hoeft P, *et al*. Prognostic value of serum cardiac troponin I and T in chronic dialysis patients: a 1-year outcomes analysis. Am J Kid Dis 1997; 29: 399-403.

[76] McLaurin MD, Apple FS, Falahati A, Murakami MM, Miller EA, Sharkey SW. Cardiac troponin I and creatine kinase-MB mass to rule out myocardial injury in hospitalized patients with renal insufficiency. Am J Cardiol 1998; 82: 973-5.

[77] Hamm CW, Bassand JP, Agewall S, *et al*. ESCGuidelines for the management of acute coronary syndromes in patients presenting without persistent ST-segment elevation: The Task Force for the management of acute coronary syndromes (ACS) in patients presenting without persistent ST-segment elevation of the European Society of Cardiology (ESC). Eur Heart J. 2011; 32(23): 2999-3054.

[78] Steg G, James SK., Atar D *et al*. ESC Guidelines for the management of acute myocardial infarction in patients presenting with ST-segment elevation. European Heart Journal 2012; 33,2569-2619.

[79] Bristel-Myers Squibb: Eliquis prescribing information. New Jersey 08543 USA, December 2012. Available from http// www.packageinserts.bms.com/pi/pi_eliquis.pdf.

[80] Granger CB, Alexander JH, McMurray JJ, *et al*. Apixaban *versus* warfarin in patients with atrial fibrillation. NEJM 2011; 365: 981-92.

[81] Lassen MR, Gallus AS, Pineo GF,*et al*. Apixaban *versus* enoxaparin for thromboprophylaxis after knee replacement (ADVANCE-2): a randomised double-blind trial. Lancet 2010 Mar 6; 375(9717): 807-15.

[82] Alexander JH, Lopes RD, James S, *et al*. APPRAISE-2 Investigators. Apixaban with antiplatelet therapy after acute coronary syndrome. NEJM 2011; 365: 699-708.

[83] Janssen Pharmaceuticals: Xarelta prescribing information. Titusville NJ 08560 March 2013 USA. http: //www.xareltohcp.com

[84] Patel MR, Mahaffey KW, Garg J, *et al*. ROCKET AF Investigators. Rivaroxaban *versus* warfarin in nonvalvular atrial fibrillation NEJM 2011; 365: 883-891.

[85] Bauersachs R, Berkowitz SD, Brenner B *et al*. Oral rivaroxaban for symptomatic venous thromboembolism N Engl J Med 2010; 363: 2499-510.

[86]   Wong H, Nunokawa N, Song JC, *et al*. Rivaroxaban: A Direct Factor Xa Inhibitor for VTE Prophylaxis in Patients Undergoing Total Knee or Hip Replacement Surgery.' Formulary 2009; 44: 226-36.

[87]   Mega JL, Braunwald E, Wiviott SD *et al*. ATLAS ACS 2-TIMI 51 Investigators. Rivaroxaban in patients with a recent acute coronary syndrome. NEJM 2012; 366: 9-19.

[88]   Stangier J, Rathgen K, Stahle H, Gansser D, Roth W. The pharmacokinetics, pharmacodynamics and tolerability of dabigatran etexilate, a new oral direct thrombin inhibitor, in healthy male subjects. Br J Clin Pharmacol 2007; 64: 292-303.

[89]   Boehringer Ingelheim Pharmaceuticals Inc.: Pradaxa Prescribing Information. Ridgefield 06877 CT USA April 2013. Available from http//www.bidocs.boehringer-ingelheim.com.

[90]   Schirmer SH, Baumhäkel M, Neuberger HR, *et al*. Novel anticoagulants for stroke prevention in atrial fibrillation: current clinical evidence and future developments. J Am Coll Cardiol 2010; 56: 2067-76.

[91]   Eriksson BI, Dahl OE, Rosencher N *et al*. Dabigatran etexilate *versus* enoxaparin for prevention of venous thromboembolism after total hip replacement: a randomised, double-blind, non-inferiority trial. Lancet, 2007; 370: 949-956

[92]   Schulman S, Kearon C, Kakkar AK, *et al*. RE-COVER Study Group. Dabigatran *versus* warfarin in the treatment of acute venous thromboembolism. NEJM 2009; 361: 2342-52.

[93]   Connolly SJ, Ezekowitz MD, Yusuf S. Dabigatran *versus* warfarin in patients with atrial fibrillation. N Engl J Med 2009; 361: 1139-51.

[94]   Oldgren J, Budaj A, Granger CB, *et al*. RE-DEEM Investigators. Dabigatran *vs*. placebo in patients with acute coronary syndromes on dual antiplatelet therapy: a randomized, double-blind, phase II trial. Eur Heart J 32; 2011: 2781-89.

[95]   Hohnloser SH, Oldgren J, Yang S, *et al*. Myocardial ischemic events in patients with atrial fibrillation treated with dabigatran or warfarin in the RE-LY (Randomized Evaluation of Long-Term Anticoagulation Therapy) trial. Circulation 2012; 125: 669.

[96]   Uchino K, Hernandez AV. Dabigatran association with higher risk of acute coronary events: meta-analysis of noninferiority randomized controlled trials. Arch Intern Med 2012 Mar 12; 172(5): 397-402.

[97]   Siller-Matula JM, Krumphuber J, Jilma B. Pharmacokinetic, pharmacodynamic and clinical profile of novel antiplatelet drugs targeting vascular diseases. Br J Pharmacol 2010; 15: 502-17.

[98]   Tricoci P, Huang Z, Held C, *et al*. TRACER Investigators. Thrombin-receptor antagonist vorapaxar in acute coronary syndromes. NEJM 2012; 366: 20-33.

[99]   O'Donoghue ML, Bhatt DL, Wiviott SD, *et al*. LANCELOT-ACS Investigators. Safety and tolerability of atopaxar in the treatment of patients with acute coronary syndromes: the lessons from antagonizing the cellular effects of Thrombin–Acute Coronary Syndromes Trial. Circulation 2011; 123: 1843-53.

[100]   Costopoulos C, Niespialowska-Steuden M, Kukreja N, Gorog DA. Novel oral anticoagulants in acute coronary syndrome. Int J Cardiol 2013 Sep 10; 167(6): 2449-55.

CHAPTER 8

Infectious Pathogens in Acute Atherosclerosis

Gulfem Ece*

Izmir University School of Medicine, Medicalpark Hospital, Department of Medical Microbiology, Yeni Girne Boulevard, No: 1825, Karsiyaka, Izmir, Turkey

Abstract: Coronary artery disease is the cause of 20% of deaths worldwide, increasing up to 50% in developed countries. Atherosclerosis is a multifactorial disease that is strongly affected by inborn and acquired risk factors. It has predisposing factors such as hypercholesterolemia, hypertension, diabetes mellitus or smoking. The contribution of infection to atherosclerosis is still a challenge. Infectious agents can aggrevate plaque rupture, and cause acute myocardial infarction and death. Atherosclerosis is a chronic inflammatory process. Various bacterial and viral pathogens have been considered as a cause for inflammation of the vascular wall which leads to atherosclerosis. *C. pneumoniae*, *H. pylori*, influenza A virus, Hepatitis C virus, Cytomegalovirus, and human immunodeficiency virus (HIV) are related to atherosclerosis. This chapter is about the potential role of these infectious pathogens in acute atherosclerosis.

Keywords: Coronary artery disease, acute mycocardial infarction, atherosclerosis, bacterial pathogens, *C. pneumoniae*, coagulation, Cytomegalovirus, endothelial cell, foam cell, gp120, *H. pylori*, Hepatitis C virus, HIV, infectious pathogens, inflammation, influenza A virus, macrophage, plaque rupture, proinflammatory cytokines, viral agents.

INTRODUCTION

Atherosclerosis is a leading cause of coronary heart disease and stroke, and leads to 25% of all deaths in the United States. It is a process that is caused by the accumulation of fatty substances, cholesterol, cellular waste products, calcium and other substances inside of an artery. This is called plaque. Rupturing plaques may obstruct blood flow or travel to any other part of the body. This situation can cause a heart attack. The decrease in blood supply to the arms can gradually lead to gangrene [1]. There are also important and additive risk factors such as age, gender, hyperlipidaemia, hypertension, smoking, diabetes mellitus and obesity [2,

---

*Corresponding author Gulfem Ece: Izmir University School of Medicine, Medicalpark Hospital, Department of Medical Microbiology, Yeni Girne Boulevard, No:1825, Karsiyaka, Izmir, Turkey; Tel: +905322731711; Fax: +902323995070; E-mail: gulfem.ece@izmir.edu.tr

3]. Monocytes and macrophages are also part of atheromatous plaques. Elevated levels of the acute phase proteins, fibrinogen and C-reactive protein and pro-inflammatory cytokines are related with an increased risk of cardiovascular events. Chronic infection may be a factor in inflammatory markers [4]. The task of infection in atherosclerosis is still a debate. There is also the issue that infection can aggrevate plaque rupture, and cause acute myocardial infarction and death [5].

The relationship between infection and atherosclerosis was first shown in 1978, and various infectious patogens have been investigated since that time [6]. Minick *et al.*, indicated that Marek's disease virus, an avian herpesvirus, caused atherosclerotic-like lesions in multiple arteries of chickens and that infection of smooth muscle cells by this virus caused cholesterol accumulation [7, 8].

Atherosclerosis is a chronic inflammatory process and a large spectrum of bacterial and viral pathogens have contributed to the inflammation of the vascular wall that leads to atherosclerosis [9]. *C. pneumoniae, P. gingivalis, H. pylori,* influenza A virus, Hepatitis C virus, Cytomegalovirus (CMV), and human immunodeficiency virus are related to atherosclerosis. In some cases, it was was demonstrated that the infectious pathogens exist in these plaques and viable organisms can be isolated. Besides, other situations, the relationship can be supported by biomarkers, and in HIV infection the reason is because of using of anti-retroviral therapy [10]. Possible mechanisms of atherosclerosis caused by infectious pathogens are shown in Table **1**.

Table 1: Possible mechanisms of infectious agents causing atherosclerosis

Infectious Agent	Mechanism of Atherosclerosis
Cytomegalovirus (CMV)	Causes cellular proliferation and inhibits apoptosis of infected smooth muscle cells, and thus contribute to an increase in the mass of arteriosclerotic lesions
H.pylori	Affects clotting mechanisms
Human Immunodeficiency virus (HIV)	Envelope protein, gp120, stimulates human arterial smooth-muscle cells to express tissue factor, the initiator of the coagulation cascade.
Hepatitis C virus (HCV)	Stimulates macrophage foam cell formation and leads to immune system activation
Influenza A virus	Affects inflammatory and coagulation pathways, and this leads to destabilisation of atherosclerotic plaques
C. pneumoniae	Increases expression of adhesion molecules, tissue factor, plasminogen activator inhibitor

Chronic infections, like periodontitis, chronic bronchitis and infection with *Helicobacter pylori, Chlamydia pneumoniae* or Cytomegalovirus are linked to atherosclerosis. The aggregate burden of chronic or past infections is linked to the risk of stroke [11] (Fig. **1**).

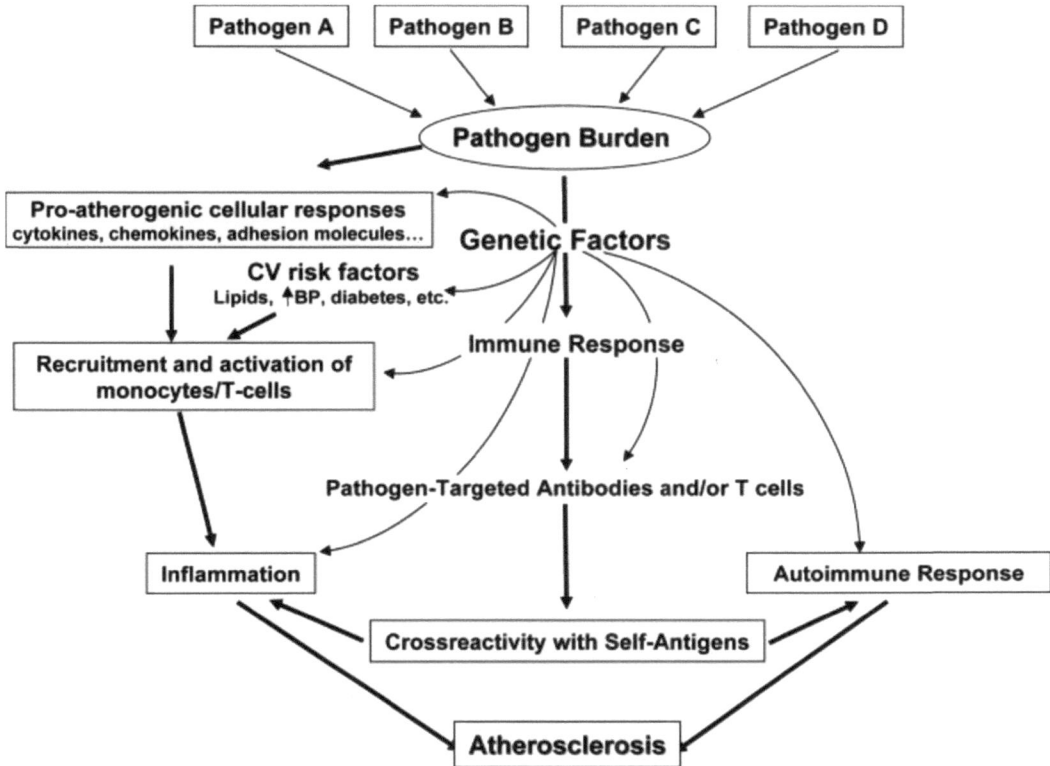

Figure 1: Multiple mechanisms by which infection may contribute to atherosclerosis development and course [12].

C. pneumoniae

The first data that *Chlamydia pneumoniae* had a relation with atherosclerosis and coronary heart disease was reported in 1988. Saikku *et al.*, reported that Finnish men with coronary heart disease more frequently had more *C. pneumoniae* antibodies than control subjects [13].

C. pneumonia infection increases expression of adhesion molecules, tissue factor, plasminogen activator inhibitor and also facilitates atherosclerosis [14, 15]. *C. pneumoniae* is active in all steps of atherosclerosis, varying from the initial inflammatory lesion to plaque rupture. It can penetrate to the vascular structure during local inflammation of the lower respiratory tract, while the organism is around the body in blood mononuclear cells [16].

It can infect vascular endothelial cells *in vitro*, and triggers secretion of pro-inflammatory cytokines and the expression of leucocyte adhesion molecules that leads to inflammation in the vessel wall and initiates lesion formation [17]. *C. pneumoniae* may provide macrophages phagocyte high level of native LDL and turn into foam cells. Besides, Chlamydial lipopolysaccharide and chlamydial heat-shock protein 60 can induce oxidation of LDL within the neointima, and cause *C. pneumoniae* to induce foam cell formation [18] (Fig. **2**).

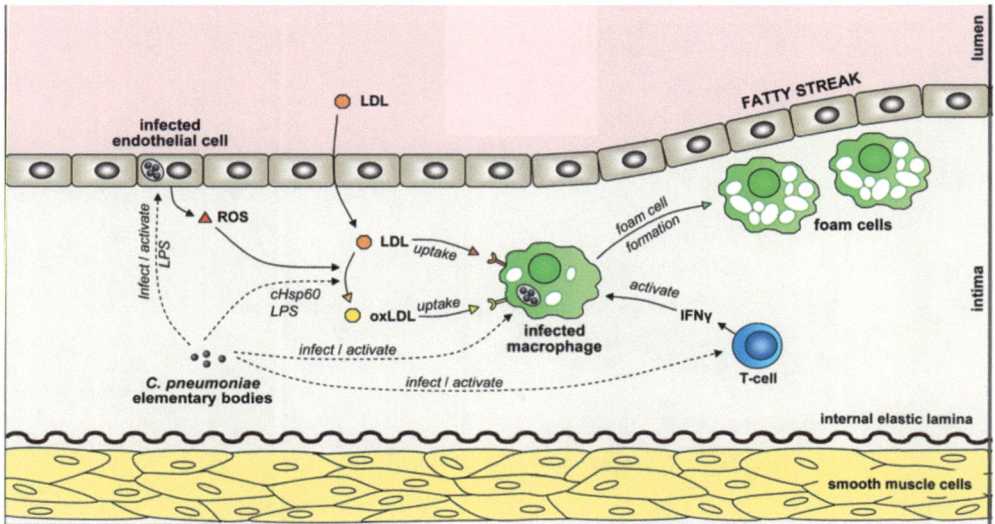

Figure 2: *C. pneumoniae* stimulates the uptake of oxidative LDL and also native LDL, and causes macrophages to turn into foam cells [17].

H. pylori

H. pylori is a Gram-negative spiral bacterium and causes gastritis and peptic ulcer disease. It has an effect on clotting mechanisms [19]. It influences the development of atherosclerotic changes in coronary arteries [20]. It may lead to an increased risk of arteriosclerosis by an autoimmune process by heat shock proteins [21]. This bacterium also induces the development of atherosclerotic changes in coronary arteries by their products such as cytokines, endotoxins, cytotoxins and other virulence factors on coronary endothelium. Besides this infectious pathogen activates acute phase responses and procoagulant hemostatic factors triggering atherosclerosis [22].

Gastric infection can stimulate the synthesis of acute phase reactants and iniates immune mechanisms by cross-reacting antibodies to *H. pylori* and heat shock protein [23-25].

The detection of *H. pylori* DNA in atheromatous plaque material isolated from coronary arteries and its relation to CagA and clinical symptoms could be an evidence for infection in the development of unstable angina because of coincident coronary artery disease triggered by a local inflammatory process [22].

Influenza A Virus

During influenza epidemics people with underlying diseases such as cardiovascular disease are especially at risk [26]. Influenza virus is related with acute coronary syndrome and induction of myocardial infarction [27]. The influenza virus affects inflammatory and coagulation pathways, and this leads to destabilisation of atherosclerotic plaques and as a result coronary artery obstruction takes place. This is the main reason for acute myocardial infarction [28, 29].

Influenza infection improves the progression of atherosclerosis and aggrevates acute coronary syndrome. Some of the studies showed the association between influenza virus infection and acute coronary syndrome [30].

The virus triggers an inflammatory and procoagulant stimulus and transiently changes endothelial function [31, 32].

Influenza virus stimulates acute myocardial infarction and cardiovascular death, and influenza vaccines may be effective for decreasing the risk of cardiac events in patients with cardiovascular disease [33].

Hepatitis C Virus

Chronic hepatitis C virus (HCV) infection is prevalent globally and approximately 170 million people are affected. HCV infection can end up with cirrhosis ascites, variceal bleeding, encephalopathy and hepatocellular carcinoma [34, 35]. The infection is related to systemic inflammation and metabolic complications that might lead patients to atherosclerosis [36, 37]. Hepatitis C virus can lead to development and progression of carotid atherosclerosis. It can stimulate macrophage foam cell formation and lead to immune system activation. This can potentiate the immune inflammatory reaction causing atherosclerosis [38].

There also have been studies on an association between HCV positivity and coronary artery disease and besides between HCV core protein and carotid atherosclerosis [39-41]. Also HCV-RNA was detected in human carotid plaques [42].

Cytomegalovirus (CMV)

Cytomegalovirus (CMV) is a common viral agent that is a member of *Herpesviridae* family [43]. During the acute phase of CMV infection, many cell types in organ systems may be infected. These cell types can be endothelial cells, epithelial cells, smooth muscle cells, fibroblasts, neuronal cells, hepatocytes, trophoblasts, monocytes, macrophages and dendritic cells [44].

CMV is the largest of the herpesviruses. CMV infection of endothelial cells may cause cellular proliferation and inhibit apoptosis of infected smooth muscle cells, and thus contributes to an increase in the mass of arteriosclerotic lesions. Besides, individuals with this infection have impaired coronary vasodilator response [45].

CMV can create phenotypic transformation of endothelial cells from a normal anticoagulant to a procoagulant phenotype, and an increment in synthesis of tissue factor and the rate of thrombin generation and a decrease in prostacyclin and thrombomodulin formation [46].

A study found out that heart transplant recipients which are seropositive for CMV antibody had higher incidence of atherosclerosis and graft rejection in the recipient heart than CMV negative ones [47].

Various studies have indicated that CMV infection of the vessel wall affects various cells including monocytes, macrophages, smooth muscle cells and endothelial cells. This infection stimulates increased expression of endothelial adhesion molecules and changes proteolytic equilibrium in monocytes and macrophages. Infected endothelium attracts monocytes from the blood stream, and the simultaneous interaction between infected endothelial cells and monocytes makes virus transfer to migrating monocytes. Endothelial damage induces thrombin formation, inflammation and coagulation. It stimulates thrombin formation and besides it may interact with the prothrombinase protein complex and facilitate thrombin generation. Thus, infection of endothelium may significantly increase the production of thrombin. This situation of thrombosis in patients with atherosclerosis also induces thrombin-dependent proinflammatory cell activation [48].

Human Immunodeficiency Virus (HIV)

Globally, 40 million people are infected with Human Immmnunodeficiency Virus (HIV). Africa, Asia, and Latin America, have the highest rates of new infections. It is the fourth reason of mortality worldwide [49].

There are reports about acute coronary thrombotic events in patients with HIV infection. Atherosclerotic plaques within carotid arteries were detected in a large proportion of middle-aged HIV-positive individuals. It was shown that HIV envelope protein, gp120, stimulates human arterial smooth-muscle cells to express tissue factor, the initiator of the coagulation cascade. The activation of smooth muscle cells by gp120 is important in the vascular, thrombotic, and inflammatory responses to HIV [50, 51].

HIV replication and immune activation can lead to coagulation and fibrinolysis. Patients with untreated HIV infection and thrombocytopenia get worse with the progressing infection [52, 53].

Besides chronic platelet activation is present and this may trigger atherogenesis, and also increase the risk for thrombosis [54] (Fig. **3**).

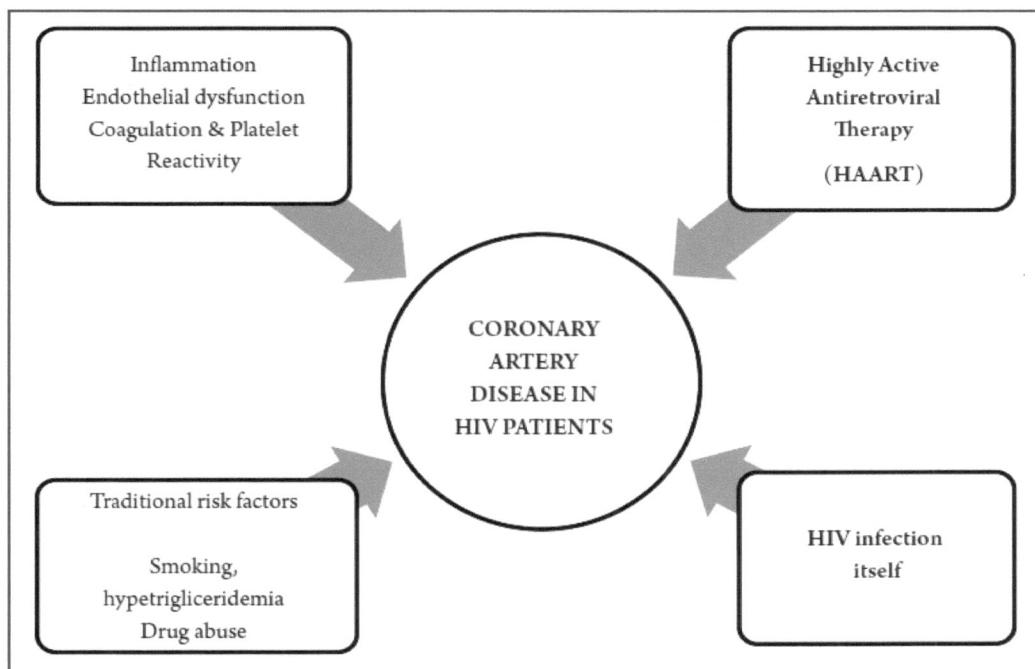

Figure3: Coronary artery disease in HIV infection [55].

Gradually people with HIV ifection start living longer due to antiretroviral therapy, and because of this cardiovascular disease has become an increasingly important cause of morbidity and mortality. But it remains doubthful if HIV infection is an additive factor to atherosclerosis independent of traditional cardiovascular risk factors. In a study, more than 400 HIV seropositive patients without previous cardiovascular disease in the FRAM (Fat Redistribution and Metabolic Change in HIV Infection) study were compared with HIV (-) ones in the MESA (Multi-Ethnic Study of Atherosclerosis) cohort study. HIV infection was accompanied by more extensive atherosclerosis as measured by intima medial thickness. The association of HIV infection with intima media thickness was similar to cardiovascular disease risk factors, such as smoking [56].

The decreased intracellular glutatione and plasma cysteine observed in HIV patients may also be due to chronic oxidative stress and this may lead to the progression of the disease. N-acetyl-cysteine administration to AIDS patients improves their hematological profile, glutatione content and survey [57].

CONCLUSION

Atherosclerosis is the leading cause of coronary heart disease and stroke. Chronic infection may be a factor in inflammatory markers. Infection can aggrevate plaque rupture, and cause acute myocardial infarction and death. The task of infection in atherosclerosis is still a debate. It is stil not clear whether chronic inflammation or the the pathogen increase the incidence of myocardial infarction. Further studies are required to prove this data.

ACKNOWLEDGEMENTS

Declared none.

CONFLICT OF INTEREST

The authors confirm that this chapter contents have no conflict of interest.

REFERENCES

[1]   Grunfeld C, Delaney JA, Wanke C, *et al*. Preclinical atherosclerosis due to HIV infection: carotid intima-medial thickness measurements from the FRAM study. AIDS. 2009; 23(14): 1841-1849
[2]   AL-Ghamdi A, Jiman-Fatani A, El-Banna H. Role of *Chlamyia pneumoniae, Helicobacter pylori* and Cytomegalovirus in coronary artery disease. Pak J Pharm Sci 2011; 24(2): 95-101.
[3]   Yusuf, S, Hawken S, Ounpuu S. *et al*. Effect of potentially modifiable risk factors associated with myocardial infarction in 52 countries (the INTERHEART study): case-control study. Lancet 2004; 364: 937-952.
[4]   Ridker PM, Hennekens CH, Buring JE, Rifai N. C-reactive protein and other markers of inflammation in the prediction of cardiovascular disease in women. N Engl J Med 2000; 342: 836-843.
[5]   Rupprecht HJ, Blankenberg S, Bickel C, Rippin G, Hafner G, Prellwitz W, Schlumberger W, Meyer J. Impact of viral and bacterial infectious burden on long-term prognosis in patients with coronary artery disease. Circulation 2001; 104: 25-31.

[6]   Libby P, Egan D, Skarlatos S. Roles of infectious agents in atherosclerosis and restenosis: an assessment of the evidence and need for future research. Circulation 1997; 96 (11): 4095-103.

[7]   Minick CR, Fabricant CG, Fabricant J, Litrenta MM. Atheroarteriosclerosis induced by infection with a herpesvirus. Am J Pathol. 1979; 96: 673-706.

[8]   Fabricant CG, Fabricant J, Minick CR, Litrenta MM. Herpesvirusinduced atherosclerosis in chickens. Fed Proc 1983; 42: 2476 -2479.

[9]   Mitchell S.V. Elkind. Infectious burden: a new risk factor and treatment target for atherosclerosis. Infect Disord Drug Targets. 2010 April 1; 10(2): 84-90

[10]   Jiang B, Hebert VY, Khandelwal AR, Stokes KY, Dugas TR. HIV-1 antiretrovirals induce oxidant injury and increase intimamedia thickness in an atherogenic mouse model. Toxicol Lett 2009; 187: 164-171.

[11]   Armin J, Grau AJ, Urbanek C Frederick Palm F. Common infections and the risk of stroke. Nature Reviews 2012; (6): 681-694 (December 2010) | doi: 10.1038/nrneurol.2010.163

[12]   Epstein SE, Zhu J, Najafi AH, Burnett MS. Insights Into the Role of Infection in Atherogenesis and in Plaque Rupture. Circulation 2009; 119: 3133-3141.

[13]   Saikku P, Leinonen M, Mattila K, *et al*. Serological evidence of an association of a novel Chlamydia, TWAR, with chronic coronary heart disease and acute myocardial infarction. Lancet 1988; 2: 983-6

[14]   Kaukoranta-Tolvanen SS, Ronni T, Leinonen M, Saikku P, Laitinen K. Expression of adhesion molecules on endothelial cells stimulated by *Chlamydia pneumoniae*. Microb Pathog 1996; 21: 407-411.

[15]   Fong IW. Biological mechanisms and animal models. In: Infections and the cardiovascularsystem: new perspectives. New York: Kluwer Academic/Plenum Publishers, 2003: 144-9.

[16]   Yang ZP, Kuo CC, Grayston JT. Systemic dissemination of *Chlamydia pneumoniae* following intranasal inoculation in mice. J. Infect. Dis.1995; 171: 736-738.

[17]   Watson C, Alp NJ. Role of *Chlamydia pneumoniae* in atherosclerosis. Clinical Science 2008; 114, 509-531.

[18]   Kalayoglu MV, Hoerneman B, LaVerda D, Morrison SG, Morrison RP, Byrne GI. Cellular oxidation of low-density lipoprotein by *Chlamydia pneumoniae*. J. Infect. Dis 1999; 180: 780-790.

[19]   Khurshid, A, Fenske T, Bajwa T, Bourgeois K,. Vakil N. A prospective, controlled study of *Helicobacter pylori* seroprevalence in coronary artery disease. Am J Gastroenterol 1998; 93: 717-720.

[20]   Niemela S, Karttunen T, Korhonen T, *et al*. Could *Helicobacter pylori* infection increase the risk of coronary heart disease by modifying serum lipid concentrations? Heart 1996; 75: 373-375.

[21]   Claudia Stöllberger and Josef FinstererCoronary and Cerebrovascular Role of Infectious and Immune Factors in atherosclerosis. Clin Diagn Lab Immunol. 2002 March; 9(2): 207-215

[22]   Kowalski M, Pawlik M, Konturek JW,.Konturek SJ. *Helicobacter Pylori* infection in coronary artery disease. Journal of Physiology and Pharmacology 2006, 57(3): 101-111.

[23]   Mendall MA, Patel P, Ballam L, *et al*. C-reactive protein and its relation to cardiovascular risk factors: a population based cross sectional study. Br Med J 1996; 312: 1061-1065.

[24]   Murray LJ, Bamford KB, O.Reilly DP, *et al*. *Helicobacter pylori* infection: relation with cardiovascular risk factors, ischemic heart disease, and social class. Br Heart J 1995; 74: 497-501.

[25]   Birnie DH, Holme ER, McKay IC, *et al*. Association between antibodies to heat shock protein 65 and coronary atherosclerosis. Possible mechanism of action of *Helicobacter pylori* and other bacterial infections in increasing cardiovascular risk. Eur Heart J 1998; 19: 387-394.

[26]   Davis MM, Taubert K, Benin AL, *et al*. Infl uenza vaccination as secondary prevention for cardiovascular disease: a science advisory from the American Heart Association/American College of Cardiology. Circulation 2006; 114: 1549-53.

[27]   Warren-Gash C, *et al*. Influenza as a trigger for acute myocardial infarction or death from cardiovascular disease: a systematic review. Lancet Infect Dis 2009; 9: 601-610.

[28]   Madjid M, Aboshady I, Awan I, Litovsky S, Casscells SW. Infl uenza and cardiovascular disease: is there a causal relationship? Tex Heart Inst J 2004; 31: 4-13.

[29]   White HD, Chew DP. Acute myocardial infarction. Lancet 2008; 372: 570-84.

[30]   Phrommintikul A, Kuanprasert S, Wongcharoen W, Kanjanavanit R, Chaiwarith R, Sukonthasarn A. Influenza vaccination reduces cardiovascular events in patients with acute coronary syndrome. Eur Heart J. 2011; 32(14): 1730-5.

[31]   Harskamp RE, van Ginkel MW. Acute respiratory tract infections: a potential trigger for the acute coronary syndrome. Ann Med 2008; 40: 121-28.
[32]   Madjid M, Awan I, Ali M, Frazier L, Casscells W. Influenza and atherosclerosis: vaccination for cardiovascular disease prevention. Expert Opin Biol Ther 2005; 5: 91-96.
[33]   Warren-Gash C, Smeeth L, Hayward AC. Influenza as a trigger for acute myocardial infarction or death from cardiovascular disease: a systematic review. Lancet Infect Dis 2009; 9: 601-10.
[34]   Lauer GM, Walker BD.Hepatitis C virus infection. N Engl JMed 2001; 345: 41-52.
[35]   Flamm SL. Chronic hepatitis C virus infection. JAMA 2003; 289: 2413-2417.
[36]   Volzke H, Schwahn C, Wolff B, *et al*. Hepatitis B and Cvirus infection and the risk of atherosclerosis in a general population. Atherosclerosis 2004; 174: 99-103.
[37]   Forde KA, Haynes K, Troxel AB, Trooskin S, Osterman MT, Kimmel SE, Lewis JD, V. Lo Re. Risk of myocardial infarction associated with chronic hepatitis C virus infection: a population-based cohort study. Journal of Viral Hepatitis 2012; 19(4): 271-277.
[38]   Espinola-Klein C, Rupprecht HJ, Blackenberg S *et al*. Impact of infectious burden on progression of carotid atherosclerosis. Stroke 2002; 33: 2581-2586.
[39]   Vassalle C, Masini S, Bianchi F, Zucchelli GC. Evidence for association between hepatitis C virus seropositivity and coronary artery disease. Heart 2004; 90: 565-6.
[40]   Ishizaka Y, Ishizaka N, Takahashi E, *et al*. Association between hepatitis C virus core protein and carotid atherosclerosis. Circ J 2003; 67: 26-30.
[41]   Ishizaka N, Ishizaka Y, Takahashi E, *et al*. Association between hepatitis C virus seropositivity, carotid-artery plaque, and intima-media thickening. Lancet 2002; 359: 133-5.
[42]   Boddi M, Abbate R, Chellini B, *et al*. HCV infection facilitates asymptomatic carotid atherosclerosis: preliminary report of HCV RNA localization in human carotid plaques. Dig Liver Dis 2007; 39: S55-60.
[43]   Mocarski ES, Shenk T, Pass R. Cytomegaloviruses. In Fields Virology. Volume 2. Fifth edition. Edited by: Knipe D, Howley P. Lippincott Williams and Wilkins; 2007: 2701-2772.
[44]   Sinzger C, Jahn G: Human cytomegalovirus cell tropism and pathogenesis. Intervirology 1996, 39: 302-319.
[45]   Epstein SE, Zhou YF, Zhu J. Infection and atherosclerosis. Emerging mechanistic paradigms. Circulation1999; 100: e20-e28.
[46]   van Dam-Mieras MC, Muller AD, van Hinsbergh VW, Mullers WJ, Bomans PH, Bruggeman CA. The procoagulant response of cytomegalovirus infected endothelial cells. Thromb Haemost. 1992; 68: 364 -370.
[47]   Grattan MT, Moreno-Cabral CE, Starnes VA, *et al*. Cytomegalovirusinfection is associated with cardiac allograft rejection and atherosclerosis. JAMA. 1989; 261(24): 3561-3566
[48]   Popović M, Smiljanić K, Dobutović B, Syrovets T, Simmet T, Isenović ER. Human cytomegalovirus infection and atherothrombosis. J Thromb Thrombolysis. 2012 Feb; 33(2): 160-72.
[49]   Pedersen NC, Ho E, Brown ML, Yamamoto JK. Isolation of a T-lymphotropic virus from domestic cats with an immunodeficiency-like syndrome. Science. 1987; 235: 790-793
[50]   Depairon, M., S. Chessex, P. Sudre, N. Rodondi, N. Doser, J. P. Chave, W. Riesen, P. Nicod, R. Darioli, A. Telenti, and V. Mooser, with The Swiss HIV Cohort Study. 2001. Premature atherosclerosis in HIV-infected individuals: focus on protease inhibitor therapy. AIDS 15: 329-334.
[51]   Schecter, A. D., A. B. Berman, L. Yi, A. Mosoian, C. M. McManus, J. W.Berman, M. E. Klotman, and M. B. Taubman. HIV envelope gp120 activates human arterial smooth muscle cells. Proc. Natl. Acad. Sci. 2001; 98: 10142-10147.
[52]   Blann AD, Seigneur M, Constans J, *et al*. Soluble P-selectin, thrombocytopenia and von Willebrand factor in HIV infected patients. Thromb Haemost 1997; 77: 1221-2.
[53]   Seigneur M, Constans J, Blann A, *et al*. Soluble adhesion molecules and endothelial cell damage in HIV infected patients. Thromb Haemost 1997; 77: 646.
[54]   Karmochkine M, Ankri A, Calvez V, *et al*. Plasma hypercoagulability is correlated to plasma HIV load. Thromb Haemost 1998; 80: 208-9.
[55]   Cerrato E, D'Ascenzo F, Biondi-Zoccai G, *et al*. Acute coronary syndrome in HIV patients: from pathophysiology to clinical practice. Cardiovasc Diagn Ther 2012; 2: 50-55.
[56]   Grunfeld C, Delaney JA, Wanke C, *et al*. Preclinical atherosclerosis due to HIV infection: carotid intima-medial thickness measurements from the FRAM study. AIDS. 2009; 23(14): 1841-1849

[57]   Guilford T, Morris D, Gray D, Venketaraman V. Atherosclerosis: pathogenesis and increased occurrence in individuals with HIV and Mycobacterium tuberculosis infection. HIV/AIDS - Research and Palliative Care 2010: 2 211-218.

152

Subject Index

A

abciximab	125
adiponectin	14
alternative drugs	97
antiphospholipid syndrome	72
anti-thrombin III deficiency	70
antiplatelet resistance	79
apixaban	132
argatroban	127
aspirin	106,123
aspirin resistance	81
atherosclerosis and vulnerable plaque	3
atherosclerosis-related biomarkers	12
atherothrombosis-related biomarkers	13
atopaxar	134

B

biochemical characterization	28
biomarkers in atherosclerosis	5
bivalirudin	127

C

C. pneumoniae	143
cangrelor	113
carbohydrates	40
cardiovascular risk factors	73
chemokines and chemokine receptors	9
cilastazol	125
circulating soluble cd40 ligand	10
clinical approach and practice guidelines	128
clopidogrel	108, 124
clopidogrel dose increase	95
clopidogrel resistance	89
complement reactive protein	7
complex formation with fvIIa	36
cysteines and disulfides	43
cytomegalovirus (CMV)	146

D

dabigatran	133
definition	89
detecting aspirin resistance	84
dimerization	38
direct thrombin inhibitors	127
dysfibrinogenemias	74

E

epidemiology	84
etiology	84
etiology and epidemiology	89
extracellular mediators and biomarkers	11

F

Factor Xa Inhibitors	128
fibrinolysis	64
fondaparinux	128

G

glycoprotein IIb/IIIa inhibitors	125
glycoprotein IIb/IIIa resistance	98

H

H. pylori	144
hemostasis: general principles	59
hepatitis C virus	145
human immunodeficiency virus (HIV)	146
hyperhomocysteinemia	72

I

indirect thrombin inhibitors	126
influenza a virus	145
interleukin-18	9
interleukin-6	8

L

lipoprotein-associated phospholipase a	2, 12
low molecular weight heparins (lmwhs)	127

M

management	88
matrix metalloproteinases	11
membrane-dependent activity	34
microparticles	14
myeloperoxidase	8

N

non-specific inflammatory biomarkers	7
novel drugs	132

O

osteopontin and osteoprotegerin	11
other biomarkers	14
other roles of tissue factor	44
oxidized low-density lipoprotein	12

P

p2y12 inhibitors	108
platelet p2y12 receptor blockers	124
posttranslational modifications	39
prasugrel	111, 124
primary hemostasis	61
protease-activated receptor antagonists	115
protein S and C deficiency	71
prothrombin gene mutations	73

R

recurrent thromboembolism	67
risk factors for VTE	69
rivaroxaban	133
role in blood coagulation	34

S

secondary hemostasis	63

Serum Heat-Shock Protein 27 (HSP27)	15
soluble adhesion molecules	10
Soluble CD36	13

T

thromboxane A2 inhibitors	106
ticagrelor	112, 125
ticlopidine	108
tissue factor	14
tissue factor structure and coagulation	23
troponins (tn)	15
tumor necrosis factor-alpha	9

U

unfractionated heparin (ufh)	126

V

vascular endothelium	60
von Willebrand factor	13
vorapaxar	115, 133

www.ingramcontent.com/pod-product-compliance
Lightning Source LLC
Chambersburg PA
CBHW041710210326
41598CB00007B/595